Fluoride
Drinking Ourselves
to Death?

Fluoride
Drinking Ourselves to Death?

Barry A. Groves

Newleaf

Newleaf
an imprint of
Gill & Macmillan Ltd
Hume Avenue
Park West
Dublin 12
with associated companies throughout the world
www.gillmacmillan.ie

© 2001 Barry A. Groves
0 7171 3274 9
Index compiled by Susan Williams
Print origination by Carole Lynch
Printed by ColourBooks Ltd, Dublin

A catalogue record is available for this book
from the British Library.

3 5 4

Dedication

This book is dedicated to the memory of Dr John Yiamouyiannis (1943–2000), a man of true honour and integrity, who died suddenly on Sunday, 8 October 2000. 'Dr Y', as he was known to his friends, worked tirelessly for many years to expose the poor science supporting fluoridation. He will be remembered both as one of that rare breed of scientists who have the courage and commitment to oppose scientific truth to political power and as one of the most brilliant scientists of the past century.

Acknowledgements

I must acknowledge the huge amount of work done over the last half-century by men and women dedicated to the search for truth. In many cases those who have spoken against fluoride have had their lives and careers ruined for blowing the whistle on fluoride or for discovering its adverse effects and then daring to publish their findings. It is to mankind's benefit that, despite incurring the wrath of their peers, they have not been cowed by the fluoride industry but have continued to tell the truth.

In writing this book, I have received help and borrowed heavily from many of the workers in this field. I cannot mention them all, and it is probably not fair to mention specific names, as all have played a part. But I must mention two who have guided me most on a personal level. The first is Jane Jones, Campaign Director of Britain's National Pure Water Association. A veritable fount of information, she fed me prodigious amounts of e-mail with the latest news. George Glasser is the other. His work in Florida has been invaluable. His investigative work in the field of pollution has been of immense help. The Florida 'sunshine laws' require public access to e-mails coming from public bodies. George has used this legal right to great effect to follow what was going on in the pro-fluoride camp.

Lastly, I should mention my wife, Monica, who did not see me for most of the days when I should have been helping around the house or garden and who read and reread this work ad nauseam – when, I'm sure, she would have preferred to be doing something else.

Contents

Foreword

Barry Groves has performed a considerable service to society by producing a clearly written book, which summarises much of the scientific evidence available on the vexed question of the fluoridation of public drinking water supplies. The format of the book is based on a circular notice sent to UK dentists by the British Fluoridation Society (BFS), which detailed a series of questions that might be posed by patients and provides suggested answers to those questions. Barry Groves takes each question and the BFS answer in turn as the basis of a series of short chapters which then present what is known and published about each topic. This juxtaposition serves to put in stark relief the apparent evasive nature or clear bias of many of the BFS's suggested responses.

What are the most important questions? Readers of this book will find that the science underpinning the widespread introduction of drinking water fluoridation, with the claim that it reduces dental decay, appears decidedly thin and shaky. For instance, the data presented shows that there are many examples of dental decay rates being higher in fluoridated than in non-fluoridated areas.

There are relatively few countries in the world that use fluoridation: the USA (where it all started) and some mainly English speaking countries across the globe. In many other countries it is simply against the law to contemplate the mass medication of a whole population with a substance that everyone, even the protagonists, admit has the potential to be toxic at certain doses. A major consideration about fluoride is that the margin of safety for fluoride is about 100 times less than that tolerated for drinking water pollutants. The industrial source of the actual fluorosilicates used to fluoridate and their potential contamination with toxic metals is thoroughly covered in the book.

What other therapeutic prophylactic substance has ever been allowed to be administered to patients, unsupervised, with no control over consumption and no recommendation for dose? Fluoride is recognised as a cumulative toxic substance and there is considerable scientific evidence to show that a proportion of the population is liable to consume more fluoride than is advisable. This can lead, amongst other conditions, to osteoporosis. Since the concept of fluoridating public water supplies was introduced we have become exposed to many other sources, through fluoridated dentifrices, tablets, and dental treatments, which has exacerbated the problem. In addition, for any drug that has ever been produced, there is a minority of the population who, because of their genetic make up, are peculiarly susceptible to its toxic properties. Furthermore there are periods, such as foetal life, infancy and extreme old age, when the body's ability to detoxify substances and excrete them are less than optimal. It appears that few considerations for such vulnerabilities in water fluoridation have been made.

Whatever the merits of the case, and you can judge those for yourselves, I am personally opposed in principle to the mass medication of whole populations. There is no shortage of products containing fluoride for people to be able to make an informed choice on their own behalf and that of their families. In addition there are no overwhelming arguments for the necessity of such treatment. This combined with the genetic susceptibility of some, as outlined above, makes the whole proposition subject to question on an ethical basis, as discussed in this book.

The book contains a number of accounts of actions that have been taken against dentists and academics who have had the temerity to question the wisdom of mass fluoridation. There would appear to have been clear violations of academic freedom. With a majority of young academics appointed to short term contracts, this is something that should exercise the minds of all those who value the importance of freedom and independence of thought amongst scientists. If academic freedom is ever allowed to be strangled then the type of data that has made the writing of this book possible will become very scarce.

I hope that you will enjoy this book, which must be regarded as essential reading for those who wish to enter an informed debate on this topic. As a microscopist who has had a research interest in the formation and build up of dental plaque and a toxico-pathologist with an interest in the effect of toxic substances on development, I have found this volume to be in turn informative, readable and thought provoking. When you have finished reading, if you come to the same conclusion, recommend it to others!

Dr C Vyvyan Howard MB, ChB, PhD, FRCPath
Toxico-Pathologist

Introduction

Fluoride is more toxic than lead and only marginally less toxic than arsenic.
Clinical Toxicology of Commercial Products, 5th edition

I cannot pretend to be an expert on the matter [fluoridation], but from what I read, it seems to be better, rather than worse, for people's health.
UK Prime Minister, Tony Blair, Prime Minister's Questions, *Hansard*, 6 May 1998

If someone were to tell you that you were being subjected to a known poison, without your consent, that the substance could lead to an increased risk of cancer and osteoporosis, and that it was used as a commercial rat poison, you would probably think they were mad. And if they averred that this medication was being administered today with the full knowledge and co-operation of government and the medical profession, you would be sure they were mad. Yet this is what is happening to millions of people in Britain, Ireland and other countries today, for that poison is fluoride.

For nearly fifty years, governments and media have been telling us that fluoride reduces dental cavities, especially in children. It is put in toothpaste, given to children in pill form, used as a gel on children's teeth, and, even though it frequently occurs naturally, the law allows water companies to add fluoride to water supplies whenever an Area Health Authority asks them to. In Ireland and some other countries, it is now quite difficult, if not impossible, to avoid fluoride.

It may come as a surprise, therefore, that although an impressive list of health, dental and regulatory organisations in Britain and Ireland (see Table 1) advocate water fluoridation

Association for Public Health

Association of Directors of Public Health Medicine

British Association for Community Child Health

British Association for the Study of Community Dentistry

British Dental Association

British Dental Health Foundation

British Dental Hygienists' Association

British Fluoridation Society

British Medical Association

British Society for Paediatric Dentistry

British Society of Dentistry for the Handicapped

Faculty of Dental Surgery of the Royal College of Surgeons of England

Faculty of General Dental Practitioners (UK) of the Royal College of Surgeons
of England

Faculty of Public Health Medicine of the Royal College of Physicians of the
United Kingdom

FDI World Dental Federation

Health Education Authority

Health Promotion Wales

Help The Aged

MENCAP

National Dental Health Education Group

NHS Confederation

NHS Consultants' Association

Oral Health Promotion Research Group

Patients Association

Public Health Alliance

Royal Society of Health

Scottish Association for Community Child Health

Socialist Health Association

Unison Health Care

*Table 1. Organisations that advocate water fluoridation in
the UK*

and actively campaign for its wider use, they represent very much a minority opinion within the scientific community; and that no country in continental Europe and only a handful of countries worldwide fluoridate their water supplies to any great extent. In other words, most have not been convinced by the pro-fluoridation lobby, even though the supposed benefits and safety of fluoride are promoted as 'incontrovertible'.

Industrial waste

The fluoride put in drinking water has never been shown to be safe. Suggested adverse effects of ingesting fluoride include dental and skeletal fluorosis, kidney disease, genetic mutations, birth defects and cancer. An acrimonious argument about whether or not fluoride should be added to drinking water with the aim of reducing dental decay has raged for half a century. For fluoride has another side that governments never mention. The 'fluorides' put in public drinking water and toothpastes are toxic industrial wastes: hazardous pollutants that, under circumstances other than water fluoridation, are very strictly controlled.

This fact has raised concern amongst health risk assessment scientists at the United States Environmental Protection Agency (EPA), who have helped draw attention to the fact that the only other place these chemicals can legally be disposed of is in a hazardous waste facility. Dr William Hirzy, senior vice-president of the trade union that represents professionals working at the EPA headquarters in Washington, DC, pointed out: '[I]f this stuff gets out into the air, it's a pollutant; if it gets into the river, it's a pollutant; if it gets into the lake, it's a pollutant; but if it goes right straight into your drinking water system, it's not a pollutant. That's amazing!'[1]

Amazing, but true.

But if overexposure to fluoride were admitted to be harmful, the impact on industry would be catastrophic:

companies would be faced with enormous bills for the disposal of this toxic waste, since fluoride is one of the most toxic substances known. Government knows about it too. If word got out (as it is doing), public health services that promote fluoridation, such as the National Health Service (NHS) in Britain, could face claims for compensation that could bankrupt them. Thus, industry and government have a powerful motive for claiming that fluoride is safe.

Fluoridation by stealth?

In 1998 the British New Labour government published a consultation paper, *Saving Lives: Our Healthier Nation*. It highlighted four priorities for improving health in Britain: heart disease and stroke, accidents, cancer, and mental health. But in the heart of the document, buried between 'an integrated transport policy' and 'tough measures on crime', are two paragraphs on fluoridation of drinking water.[2] Their disguised position may not be accidental. Frank Dobson, then Secretary of State for Health, was reported in *The Dentist* (July/August 1998) to have told officials that he intended to 'push forward' with fluoridation in the coming White Paper and, if necessary, to do so by 'subtle means'.[3]

The consultation paper said that it recognised 'the strongly held views on the issue of water fluoridation' and welcomed 'ideas on how best to test public opinion'. But surely public opinion should not decide this issue. Whether a chemical should be fed indiscriminately to the whole population with the sole purpose of altering the chemical composition of body tissues is, surely, a medical question. Is 'the public' medically qualified to take such a decision?

Only a crank would want a clean water supply

Research conducted in countries where fluoridation is not practised, and where public health officials are not committed to fluoridation, is unbiassed. It is largely in these countries that fluoride's detrimental effects have been exposed. In countries where fluoridation is practised, the reverse has been true. Over-zealous proponents have denied all evidence of harm that has come from the other countries, they have stopped scientific research, and they have stifled debate. In Britain, as in the only other countries to fluoridate their water to any extent (Ireland, the USA, New Zealand, Canada and Australia), the fluoride dispute has adversely affected both the funding that should have been devoted to studying the long-term effects of fluoride exposure, and the quality and type of research conducted. The debate, which has now continued for more than half of the twentieth century, has become acrimonious. Proponents reject as clinically insignificant every study that casts doubt on the safety of fluoridation: the adverse effects, they say, are attributable to something other than fluoride, or are irrelevant; while those who oppose fluoridation are vilified as scare-mongers, quacks and fluorophobes.

The following is a good example of such denigration. In 1996 Frances Frech, an American opposed to fluoridation, noted in a letter to the dental/public health listserv on the Internet, that the *Journal of Public Health Dentistry*, no less, had said:

> 84 per cent of 17-year-olds have had tooth decay with an average of 11 affected surfaces . . . black, low-income, and Native American children, respectively, have 65 percent, 91 percent, and 265 per cent more untreated tooth decay than their peers.[4]

Frech pointed out that

> ALL (not some, not most, ALL) Native American reservations are fluoridated by order of the US Public Health Service . . . Fluoride, then, whether safe or not, is clearly NOT very effective IF at all.[5]

With this, Frech challenged the proponents of fluoridation to a debate.

Dr Michael Easley has a PhD in dentistry from Ohio State University and an MPH (Master of Public Health) degree from Michigan State University. He is a former Director of Environmental Health and Community Safety for the Commonwealth of Kentucky. Currently, he is president and chief executive officer of International Health and Management Associates. He is the national spokesman on fluoridation for the American Dental Association and has testified on fluoridation both in the USA and in Britain. Easley answered Frech's letter on the Internet with the following attack on 7 August 1996. He warned dentists that they:

> . . . should not waste their precious time and energy dealing with these health terrorists. As you can see from Frech's propaganda, none of them know a damn thing about what they are talking about. Besides, Frech and the like make it up as they go – there is no science behind their false claims. From their perspective, that is all right though, because their twisted minds have accepted the notion that it is OK to lie, slander, libel, exaggerate, misquote, inaccurately quote, quote out of context, and invent 'truths' at the drop of a hat, in their misguided attempts to frighten the public into not accepting fluoridation. If members of this listserv would only 'surf' the net occasionally and read some of their materials, you'd see what kooks they really are.
>
> As you are all aware, there can be no legitimate debate about fluoridation because there is no scientific controversy about it – it remains safe, effective, efficient and cost-effective, regardless of what Frech and the other anti-fluoride ilk say about it. 135 million people drink fluoridated water in the US, with another 10 million drinking water that has natural fluoride levels at optimal levels. And the number is growing rapidly as we

continue to fluoridate additional cities, despite the failed attempts of the fluorophobics.

The one principle that needs to be remembered is that anti-fluoride cultists will not be dissuaded by the truth. Fluorophobics are not deserving of your efforts. Let them spew their garbage, ignore them, and go on with your discussions as if they weren't there. They have their own anti-health homepages from which they can pollute the Internet with their illogical propaganda. You won't eliminate quackery by debating with quacks – debating them here only gives them an additional forum from which to publicize their twisted logic. Spend your energy fluoridating communities. The best way to beat the anti-fluoride zealots is to fluoridate their water supply. If they don't want to drink the water, then they can buy bottled water or move to the country. The rest of their community wants and deserves fluoridation.[6]

Note the choice of words Easley uses. Calling people who simply want a wholesome water supply, uncontaminated by added medication, 'health terrorists', 'cultists' and 'quacks' is hardly the language of reasoned debate. Don't forget that Frech was quoting from a prestigious dental journal and merely asking for the issue to be debated.

But then, the second paragraph of his tirade begins: 'As you are all aware, there can be no legitimate debate about fluoridation because there is no scientific controversy about it.' Isn't there? Easley couldn't be more wrong, as this book will demonstrate. Easley cannot help but be aware of it: after all, it is his job. No, Easley doesn't *want* this subject debated.

Easley is not the first person not to want a fluoride debate. In 1961 Dr C.H. Patton, then president of the American Dental Association, told a meeting of the California Dental Association: 'I contend the subject [fluoridation] is not debatable.'[7] Four years later, the executive secretary of the ADA repeated: 'Fluoridation of drinking water is no longer a subject that is scientifically debatable.' And the following year yet another president of the ADA told a National Health Assembly: 'Fluoridation is no longer debatable in the scientific community; it should not be debatable in the political community.'[8]

Of course, if a subject cannot be debated, then any evidence, either for or against, cannot be heard. This means that those in both the dental and medical fields, who need to be aware of any adverse effects, are denied access to that information – potentially a very dangerous situation.

In a court case to decide the legality of fluoridation in Allegheny County, Pennsylvania, Judge Flaherty, formerly chairman of the Pennsylvania Academy of Sciences and now a Justice of the Supreme Court of Pennsylvania, declared: 'Prior to my hearing this case, I gave the matter of fluoridation little if any thought but I received quite an education, and noted that the proponents of fluoridation do nothing more than try to impugn the objectivity of those who oppose fluoridation.'[9]

Oppose and be damned

Vilification of those who oppose the mandatory fluoridation of drinking water is commonplace in the history of fluoridation. Voices of opposition have invariably been suppressed since its inception over half a century ago; many scientists who have spoken out against fluoridation have been fired from their jobs. It is a far from healthy story, and it still goes on today.

What should be done?

The questions hanging over the safety and effectiveness of fluoride need to be addressed as a matter of urgency. Refusing to debate this issue will not resolve the matter. Neither will burying one's head in the sand in the hope that it will go away. The safety of fluoride is firmly on the agenda, and there are many questions about fluoride that need to be answered:

1. The world witnessed a dramatic decline in the prevalence of dental caries in the twentieth century. Fluoride is frequently cited as the reason for this improvement. But caries has also declined in countries that don't fluoridate. Is the decline due to fluoride or something else?

2. The safety of the fluorides put in water have never been tested. The UK government-sponsored review of fluoridation, *Fluoridation of Drinking Water: A Systematic Review of Its Efficacy and Safety*, published in 2000, does not address this question. Nor does it look at all sources of fluoride, even though the World Health Organization says that fluorides from *all* sources must be considered before yet more are introduced into the food chain. With a recommended 1 mg per day 'required' to prevent cavities, and one cup of tea alone containing up to 7.6 mg,[10] do we really need more?

3. Or should we really be considering *removing* fluorides from our diet? This book cannot hope to cover all the thousands of studies that have been published over the past century, but it will endeavour to cover enough of both the scientific evidence on which fluoridation is based and the ethical questions that this indiscriminate mass medication raises for readers to be able to make a more informed decision about whether they want fluoride in their diet.

The British Fluoridation Society's suggested answers to issues raised by the public – and the truth

The advent of the Internet, with its millions of pages of data, has allowed the public to look at many issues connected with health, and as a consequence, people are beginning to question many of the foodstuffs and treatments available today. One result of this increasing awareness is that dentists are finding that their patients are asking more and more questions about dental treatments. Not surprisingly, those patients expect dentists to have sufficient knowledge to answer those questions.

But dentists do not know.

Some three years ago I asked my own dentist, who is a university lecturer on dentistry, what he knew about any possible adverse effects of fluoride. He replied that he knew of none, and that he left that 'to the experts'. I had expected him to be an expert.

The British Fluoridation Society (BFS) is a British government-funded limited company, composed mainly of dentists, which campaigns to put fluoride in drinking water. Because the questioning of dentists has become ever more common, the BFS recently prepared a briefing paper containing specimen questions and suggested answers, with brief background résumés, for dentists and BFS spokespeople. These questions and the BFS's suggested answers, with résumés in italics, exactly as they are presented, form the basis of the chapters in this book.

This book takes each question, its suggested answer and the brief résumé, as published by the BFS, and then answers the questions in detail with reference to published evidence. In this way it will cover issues of safety and efficacy, as well as the ethics and legality of fluoridation. It will also look at the history of fluoridation to uncover a story of arrogance and ignorance.

In addition, this book will discuss the British government-sponsored NHS review of the benefits and adverse effects of fluoridation (*Fluoridation of Drinking Water: A Systematic Review of Its Efficacy and Safety*), the results of which, published on 6 October 2000, did not show fluoride to be safe. Finally, several practical suggestions are made to enable you to avoid this iniquitous poison.

References

1. Hirzy JW. Video interview with Michael Connett. 3 July 2000.
2. *Saving lives: Our healthier nation.* London: HMSO, 1998: 3.33, 3.34.
3. Brown, Colin, 'Fluoride Boost', *The Dentist* 1998: July/August, p.55.
4. *Journal of Public Health Dentistry* 1993; 53 (1): quoted in ref. 5.
5. Frech, Frances, Challenge to Debate, http://www.sonic.net/~kryptox/letters.htm.
6. Easley, Michael, dental/public health listserv, 7 August 1996.
7. ADA head says fluoridation not debatable. *San Francisco Examiner*, 17 April 1961.
8. 1966 National Health Assembly. *Public Health Service publication no. 1552.* 1966.
9. Letter from Pennsylvania Supreme Court Justice JP Flaherty to Sir Dove-Myer Robinson the Mayor of Auckland, New Zealand, 31 July 1979.
10. BabyCenter Editorial Team with Medical Advisory Board (http://www.babycenter.com/refcap/674.html#3).

1. Water Fluoridation

What is water fluoridation?

BFS suggested answer

Water fluoridation is the most effective public health measure to prevent tooth decay. It reduces tooth decay by 50%. Water fluoridation involves adjustment of the naturally occurring fluoride in water supplies to a level which is known to be beneficial and safe, and which occurs naturally in some places – for example Hartlepool. Water fluoridation means less tooth decay for children, and older people keeping their own teeth longer.

All water supplies contain measurable amounts of fluoride. Water fluoridation is simply the adjustment of the naturally occurring fluoride to water which is known to benefit dental health – 1 part fluoride to 1 million parts water.

BFS suggested answer refuted

No laboratory test has ever shown that 1 part per million fluoride in the drinking water reduces tooth decay.
Chief Dental Officer, UK Ministry of Health and Social Security, 11 December 1980

The school bus stopped outside the village shop. Within seconds it had disgorged a large number of teenage children. They swept into the shop like locusts to strip the shelves of sweets. It was obvious that they had no thought for the harm they were doing to their health, their waistlines or their teeth. The last of these is what the British Dental Association says it is trying to protect by adding fluoride to Britain's tap water: fluoride, it says, reduces tooth decay.

At the beginning of the twentieth century, extensive dental caries (decay) was common in Britain, Ireland, the United States and most developed countries.[1] Failure to meet the minimum standard of having six opposing teeth was a leading cause of exclusion from military service in both world wars.[2] At that time there were no effective measures to prevent this disease; the most frequent treatment was tooth extraction.

Dental decay begins as soon as the first teeth start erupting and are contaminated by sugary and starchy foods. Caries is caused by bacteria. The most common bacterium implicated is *Streptococcus mutans*. The bacteria first gain attachment to the tooth surface by making a starchy 'glue'. Once attached, and given a suitable food supply, the bacteria thrive and multiply, producing colonies that we know as dental plaque. Within the plaque, millions of bacteria ferment carbohydrates (sugars and starches), producing an acid that demineralises, or eats away, the surface of the tooth, allowing in food particles and bacteria to decay the underlying material of the teeth.

Dental caries is as old as civilisation. Skulls from the period before the cultivation of grains – wheat, rice, barley, and so on – show few signs of carious (decayed) teeth. Significantly, the remains of highly cultured Sumerians of around 5,000 BC, and of the ancient Egyptian rulers wealthy enough to be buried in the pyramids, all have signs of the dental decay we see today, while those of the poorer and lower classes do not.[3] For 7,000 years, the wealthy always fared worse than the poor as far as tooth decay was concerned. But in the nineteenth century AD, and with an ever quickening pace in the twentieth, reductions in the cost of sugar led to a huge increase in the amount eaten. At the turn of the nineteenth century, we each ate, on average, about 1 kg (2 pounds) of sugar per year; now we eat around 60 kg (130 pounds). As its price dropped, sugar, and products which contain sugar, came to be regarded as necessary, indeed essential, foods. Starchy foods like white bread, polished rice and pasta were consumed in ever increasing quantities. And as a consequence, the incidence of dental caries soared in many Western countries.

As these foods are significantly cheaper than foods high in protein and fats, they are eaten in greater quantity by the poorer element in our societies, and the decay that was common in the rich, but rare among the poor, shifted to become a disease associated with poverty.

At the same time, tribes that we tend to think of as poor because they lack the material possessions we enjoy, but whose diets are restricted to meat, fish and berries – the Inuit, the Maasai, the Hunza, Siberian tribes and others – have remained caries-free. For it is sugars and refined starches alone that are the fertile breeding ground of teeth-rotting bacteria. This is illustrated vividly by a comparison between the inhabitants of the two sides of Greenland. Until about 200 years ago, all Inuit were free of dental caries. Now, those in the eastern areas with access to ice-free harbours for much of the year, and supplied with 'civilised' refined carbohydrate foods, have dental caries, while those on the largely iced-up western side of Greenland, which the traders cannot reach, are uncontaminated by the Western diet, and thus have healthy teeth.

Similarly, during World War II, the incidence of dental decay fell dramatically in occupied Denmark and Norway, where sugar was scarce, while it remained high in neutral Sweden, where sugar remained readily available.

Why fluoride?

Fluorine, a member of the halogen group of elements, is the thirteenth most common element. The most reactive of all the halogens and a deadly poison, it does not exist in nature on its own but is found only in compounds (fluorides) with other elements. Calcium fluoride is most common, as fluorine has a particularly strong affinity for calcium.

During the last years of the nineteenth century, the inhabitants of several areas of the USA had mottled teeth. Investigations showed that this mottled enamel (we now call it 'fluorosis') was caused by calcium fluoride in the drinking water. Although this condition was unsightly, it was noticed that children with it tended to have fewer decayed teeth, and it was not long before it was suggested that calcium fluoride might also be the agent responsible for conferring protection against dental caries.

Fluorides are believed to help to prevent dental caries in three ways:

- **Systemic fluoride strengthens teeth.** 'Systemic' fluoride, that is, fluoride ingested in food or water, is absorbed through the stomach and intestine into the bloodstream, where it is attracted to bones, teeth and any other calcium in the body. In young children whose teeth are growing, the interaction with the developing tooth buds initiates the replacement of the tooth enamel's normal crystalline composition ('hydroxyapatite') with a related crystal which incorporates fluoride ('fluorapatite'). As fluorapatite is believed to be more resistant to decay than the more normal hydroxyapatite, the claim is that the teeth of children who drink fluoridated water or are given fluoride supplements are less likely to develop caries. It should be borne in mind, however, that, unlike bone, tooth enamel, once fully formed, is static – it doesn't undergo metabolic changes. Thus, systemic fluoride can only be incorporated into teeth during the growing period. That is up to about the age of twelve. In Ireland we are now told that fluoridated drinking water provides a continuous supply of fluoride, via the saliva, to the tooth surface. As this denies the original systemic action hypothesis, Irish dentists have asked for, but never received, scientific evidence to support this claim.

- **Fluoride helps to remineralise teeth.** The acid produced by bacteria breaks down tooth enamel into its component chemicals. This releases the fluoride that was incorporated as the teeth developed, and it builds up in the surrounding plaque. As the concentration of fluoride in plaque increases, the bacteria's metabolisms slow down, and they consume less sugar and starch. Less consumption means less acid is produced, and less acid means less decay. It is thought that some of the dissolved minerals may be reincorporated back into the teeth.

- **Topical fluoride kills decay-causing bacteria.** All living cells, whether human, animal, vegetable or bacterial, are extremely sensitive to fluoride. At levels as low as 0.19 ppm (parts per million), fluoride interferes with certain of *S. mutans'* essential metabolic enzymes; at levels between 4 and 20 ppm, it can cause *S. mutans* to mutate; and at 20 ppm or above, it is lethal to the bacterium. Thus, fluoride, a powerful antibacterial agent, can be painted onto teeth (this is called a 'topical' application) to kill the bacteria there. Brushing teeth with a fluoridated toothpaste or a fluoride mouthwash does the same job.

The case for fluoridation of drinking water rests simply on one perceived benefit: systemic fluoride helps to prevent dental caries in children up to the age of twelve.

In the light of such evidence, major public health programmes around the world were initiated around the middle of the twentieth century to add fluoride to drinking water in areas where it was considered deficient.

In 1969, the 22nd World Health Assembly passed a resolution recommending member states to 'fluoridate water supplies where practicable in order to prevent dental caries'. It also recommended that member states study other methods of using fluorides to protect dental health. It further called upon the director-general of the World Health Organization

(WHO) to encourage research into the causation of dental caries, the fluoride content of diets, the mechanism of action of fluoride at optimal levels in drinking water and the effects of greatly excessive intake of fluoride from natural sources.

In 1974 the Executive Board, apparently noting that after five years nothing had been done, instructed the director-general to present a report to the 28th World Health Assembly in 1975.[4]

When the report was presented, the most fundamental question of what intake of fluoride, if any, was optimal had not been addressed and remained unanswered. The report contained no new research into the causes of dental decay, nor did it contain anything on the other research subjects that the 1969 assembly had proposed.

Despite these shortcomings, the 28th World Health Assembly passed a resolution, the preamble to which stated that sufficient information had already been obtained about the safety and effectiveness of the use of fluorides as a method to prevent dental caries. The assembly recommended that the WHO should 'promote approved methods for the prevention of dental caries especially by optimisation of the fluorides content of water supplies'.

Benefits of fluoride on dental caries are not apparent

We often hear statements by proponents of fluoridation to the effect that 'more than fifty years of research and practical experience have proved beyond a reasonable doubt that fluoridation is effective in preventing tooth decay. Hundreds of studies have demonstrated reduction in tooth decay of 60–70 per cent in communities with either natural or controlled fluoridation'.[5] But it is very difficult to find proof of such statements, as the most recent investigations of the status of children's teeth have found little benefit from living in a fluoridated area.

Initial studies are invalid

It was Dr H. Trendley Dean, 'the father of fluoridation', who first hypothesised that fluoridation would protect teeth from cavities. Dean also declared that it was safe and established the first trial of water fluoridation in Grand Rapids, Michigan, in 1945. Since that time, however, he has twice confessed in court that statistics from the early studies, allegedly supporting the use of fluoridation in community water systems, were invalid.[6]

In 1953 the *Journal of the American Dental Association* (*JADA*) published a comparative study of tooth decay in 12- to 14-year-olds in six Arizona cities. It found no reduction in tooth decay due to fluoridation.[7] In 1955, *JADA* published a second study.[8] This compared the teeth of children in Cameron, Texas, where the water contained 0.4 ppm natural fluoride, with those of subjects in Bartlett, Texas, where the water contained 8 ppm fluoride. There was no difference between them.

Caries declines in *unfluoridated* areas

Dennis H. Leverett, chairman of the Department of Community Dentistry, Rochester, New York, published a table in 1982 (Table 1) demonstrating that the dramatic declines in dental caries, which had been attributed to fluoride use, had also happened in *unfluoridated* areas.[9] WHO figures confirmed this,[10] as did US National Institute for Dental Research figures for over 39,000 children from eighty-four American communities. These figures indicated no difference in DMFT (decayed, missing and filled teeth) between those who lived in fluoridated, partially fluoridated or unfluoridated areas. 'The average decay rates for all children aged 5–17 were 2.0 teeth for both fluoridated and non-fluoridated areas.'[11]

Location	Time interval	Age of subjects	Caries reduction (%)
New Zealand	1950–77	5	44
NW England	1969–80	11–12	40
Isle of Wight	1971–80	11–12	18
Brisbane	1954–77	6–14	50
Geneva, NY	1965–77	12–14	41
Brockport, NY	1952–75	12	60
Boston, MA	1950–80	5–17	40–50
Massachusetts	1968–78	—	>50
Ohio	1972–78	6–12	17

Source: From Leverett DH. *Science* 1982; 217; 26–30.

Table 1. Decline in dental caries in unfluoridated areas

The director of the Division of Dental Health Services for British Columbia in Canada showed that DMFT for both fluoridated and unfluoridated areas were falling – but the areas that had the *fewest* bad teeth were those that were *not* fluoridated.[12]

'Dutch scientists found essentially no reduction in caries when the fluoride users and non-users had been carefully matched.'[13] Higher levels of fluoride in drinking water were associated with *higher* tooth decay rates in a thirty-year Indian survey of 400,000 children.[14] And in Britain, Ministry of Health figures showed that, after eleven years of fluoridation, 14-year-old children drinking fluoridated water had an average of 6.3 decayed teeth, compared with 7.2 in unfluoridated areas – a difference of less than one tooth.[15]

The illusion that fluoride prevents dental caries

North Shields and South Shields are very similar towns on opposite sides of the River Tyne. But where South Shields' water was naturally fluoridated at 1.4 ppm, North Shields' water contained little or no fluoride. In 1948 the late Robert

Weaver, then senior medical officer to the Ministry of Education, compared the two towns and found that the amount of dental caries was the same in both. South Shields' fluoridated water, he found, merely delayed the onset of caries by about three years. Such a delay appeared to show benefits when children in fluoridated areas were compared with those of the same age in control populations, but the rate of increase in decay was the same in both groups when adults and children were included. Weaver concluded: 'I think that the most important lesson to be learned from the North and South Shields investigation is that the caries-inhibitory property of fluorine seems to be of rather short duration . . . there is in fact no very striking difference in the incidence of caries in the two towns.'[16]

In 1972, Professor Albert Schatz confirmed the illusion that fluoridation reduced caries.[17] Teeth are only damaged once they have erupted and are in contact with food. By erupting later, they have a shorter exposure, and thus less decay. In 1993 Schatz declared:

> The data clearly showed that fluoridation only delays the appearance of caries . . . Fluoridated children develop the same amount of tooth decay as their non-fluoridated counterparts over their lifetime. The only difference is that caries start developing approximately 1.2 years later.
>
> There is no economic benefit for such actions. Since fluoride does not reduce caries . . . both groups will therefore require the same amount of dental treatment. People in fluoridated areas, therefore, pay for the same amount of dental treatment plus the added cost of fluoridation.

So while it can truthfully be said that fluoride is responsible for lower rates of decay seen in fluoridated children *who are the same age* as unfluoridated children, it is not because fluoride has any beneficial action on the decay. It is merely because fluoride puts it off for a while.

Table 2 demonstrates clearly this delay: the percentage difference between the numbers of decayed teeth in children who drink fluoridated water and children who do not decreases as the children get older.

Age	Average DMFT per child		% Difference in DMFT
	Fluoride areas	Non-fluoride areas	
8	1.2	2.0	67
9	1.8	2.7	50
10	2.4	3.3	37
11	3.0	4.0	33
12	4.0	5.6	40
13	5.4	6.9	28
14	6.3	7.2	14

Source: UK Department of Health. *Fluoridation studies in the United Kingdom and the results achieved after eleven years.* London: HMSO, 1969.

Table 2. DMFT *for permanent teeth of UK children drinking fluoridated and unfluoridated water*

This flaw, which was not noticed when the very early research was done, invalidates many epidemiological surveys that purport to show that children living in fluoridated areas have less tooth decay than children of the same age living in unfluoridated areas: the assumption on which the whole case for fluoride is based.

As long ago as 1960, Lord Douglas of Barloch referred to the possible delay in the eruption of teeth, saying: 'If this is so, it is a matter of grave concern for it indicates a profound physiological change.' Yet even today, this point still has not been resolved. It is standard practice for dentists to note and record which teeth are decayed, filled or missing, whether they have been shed or extracted, and which teeth have not yet erupted, for each of their patients. Therefore, it is a very simple matter to determine, for each sex, the average number of each type of tooth, and the total number of teeth, that have erupted at each age. Yet in official British experiments, no count is made of the numbers of teeth erupted, or if it is, the data aren't published – or they are deliberately suppressed.

This delay in tooth eruption also has an unexpected adverse effect. You may assume that if decay is postponed for a year or so, this gives more time for preventative measures to be introduced and, in this way, for teeth to benefit. But this appears not to be the case. In 1997 a study carried out in Tanzania showed that dental fluorosis was much more severe when dental enamel was completed later in life.[18]

WHO says so

Fluoride proponents claim that 'over a hundred studies' prove the efficacy of fluoride. This appears to be backed by the WHO publication *Environmental Health Criteria for Fluorine and Fluorides*,[19] which was published in 1984. The scientists who wrote this gave as their reference the data displayed in a poster by Drs J.J. Murray and A.J. Rugg-Gunn in 1979.[20] This poster stated that '120 fluoridation studies from all continents showed a reduction in caries in the range of 50 to 75% for permanent teeth'. Although the WHO document doesn't say it, the poster's data obviously came from a table listing 128 pro-fluoridation studies, in a book that Murray and Rugg-Gunn had published in 1982.[21]

In 1988, Philip Sutton investigated the scientific basis for the WHO's paper and published the results in *Chemical and Engineering News*.[22] Here are his findings.

There were no controls

A table of the studies (from the Murray and Rugg-Gunn book) gave the impression that fluoridated children were compared with children who had not had fluoride treatment.

Sutton found that they weren't. That in itself diminishes the authority of the studies' results.

None of the studies allowed for bias

Assessment of the effects of fluoride depends on a visual examination of children's teeth. This calls for a subjective judgement by the examining dentists. If those dentists have an opinion on the value of fluoride, and if they know in advance which children have had fluoride and which haven't, this can have an effect on their judgement, albeit an unconscious one, such that the extent of caries in the unfluoridated children is exaggerated. To avoid this, such trials should be conducted 'blind': i.e. dentists should not know whether the children they are examining have or have not been treated with fluoride. None of these studies took steps to avoid such a bias. With these defects, the value of these studies as a basis for population-wide intervention was already precarious. Sutton found, when he delved deeper, even more disturbing aspects.

Thirty-four studies didn't exist:

- Forty-six of the listed studies actually amounted to only twenty-three. Data on deciduous and permanent teeth were listed separately, thus doubling the number of studies.

- Two studies that included data from more than one town were listed as six studies.

- Seven case reports in different years from the same study were listed as fourteen studies.

Twenty studies were about something else:

- 'The most important claim made for fluoridation is that it decreases dental caries in the permanent teeth. Contrary to the statement in that WHO book, 20 studies listed did not present any data for those teeth.'

Fifty-one were of very poor scientific quality:

- Sixteen were short reports in state dental newsletters and journals.

- Fourteen were short communications in state health departments' newsletters and bulletins.

- Eight were essentially progress reports.

- Three were personal communications.

- Two were anonymous.

- Four were original trials that had been known to be faulty for twenty-five years.[23]

- Three didn't demonstrate that fluoridation is efficacious.

- And one did not refer to fluoridated water at all.

The last twenty-three

By now Sutton had whittled what had been an impressive list of 128 studies down by over 80 per cent, leaving just 23 studies. These, like all the others, turned out to be just as suspect:

- Four could not be verified, as they could not be obtained. None was even listed in the *Index to Dental Literature* or in *Index Medicus*.

- The last nineteen studies came from fluoridated countries. Sutton found that none of them showed in a scientifically acceptable manner that fluoridation was efficacious.

Therefore, in what appears to have been a comprehensive worldwide search, Murray and Rugg-Gunn were apparently unable to locate a single study demonstrating that fluoridation was effective at either reducing or preventing dental caries. The foundation on which the WHO document and subsequent fluoridation programmes in several countries were built was as substantial as quicksand.

Sutton discovered these discrepancies merely by referring to Murray and Rugg-Gunn's table and reading their references. Why didn't the WHO panel do this?

WHO European figures do not support fluoridation

The WHO monitors decayed, missing and filled teeth regularly. Its figures, shown in Table 3, provide no support for the claim that fluoridation of drinking water helps to preserve children's teeth.

Country	Year	DMFT	Year	DMFT	% Fluoridated
Finland	1975	7.5	1991	1.2	Not fluoridated
Denmark	1978	6.4	1992	1.3	Not fluoridated
UK (GB & NI)	1973	4.7	1993	1.4	10%
Sweden	1977	6.3	1994	1.5	Not fluoridated
Netherlands	1974	6.5–8.2	1991	1.7	Not fluoridated
Ireland	**1972**	**5.4**	**1992**	**1.9**	**66%**
Switzerland	1963–75	2.3–9.9	1987–89	2.0	1 city (Basle)
France	1975	3.5	1993	2.1	Not fluoridated
Norway	1973	8.4	1991	2.3	Not fluoridated
Spain	1968–69	1.9	1993	2.3	1 plant
Germany (GDR)	1973	6.0	1994	2.5	Not fluoridated
Germany (FRG)				2.6	Not fluoridated
Belgium	1972	3.1	1991	2.7	Not fluoridated
Austria	1973	1.0–3.5	1993	3.0	Not fluoridated
Italy	1978–79	4.0–6.9	1985	3.0	Not fluoridated
Portugal	1979	4.6	1989	3.2	Not fluoridated

Source: WHO Oral Health Country/Area Profile Programme, Department of Noncommunicable Diseases Surveillance/Oral Health, WHO Collaborating Centre, Malmö University, Sweden.

Table 3. Comparison of decayed, missing and filled teeth (DMFT) in 12-year-olds in European countries

The Republic of Ireland has been fluoridated for over thirty years, but in terms of the numbers of decayed, missing and filled teeth, it ranks only sixth in Europe behind countries that are not fluoridated. And in terms of *reductions* in DMFT, which is where the benefits of fluoridation are claimed to be most pronounced, Ireland drops to seventh place behind Norway, and the next most fluoridated country, the UK, drops to sixth place.

Evidence mounts

British Columbia has the lowest rates of caries in Canada. Yet only 11 per cent of the population lives in areas with fluoridated water, compared with between 40 and 70 per cent in the rest of Canada. If that weren't enough, the lowest rates of caries are found in the areas of British Columbia that are not fluoridated at all.[24]

The largest study on fluoridation and tooth decay ever undertaken was performed in India by Drs S.P.S. and M. Teotia.[25] Looking at the teeth of over 400,000 students, they discovered a 27 per cent increase in decay with a 1 ppm fluoride increase in drinking water.

A total of 39,000 children aged five to seventeen living in eighty-four different areas were the subjects of a study by the US National Institute for Dental Research. A third of the areas studied were wholly fluoridated, a third partially fluoridated, and a third unfluoridated. Although this study cost US taxpayers some $3.6 million, its results were not published. Dr John Yiamouyiannis used the Freedom of Information Act to extract the data.[26] He found that there were no significant differences in dental decay between fluoridated and unfluoridated areas.

A University of Arizona study in 1992 found that 'the more fluoride a child drinks, the more cavities appear in the teeth'.[27]

Fluoride damages teeth

It is obvious from evidence so far that fluoride is not effective at preventing caries. Much research from many parts of the world suggests that fluoride actually damages teeth. Researchers at Tokyo Medical and Dental University compared the teeth of 20,000 students and showed clearly that students from areas with levels of fluoride greater than 0.4 ppm in the water supply had significantly more decay than those whose water contained less than 0.4 ppm.[28] Another study, conducted in Ottawa, Kansas, found that water fluoridation was a disaster: in the first three years after fluoridation, the numbers of DMFT in 5- to 6-year-old children more than doubled, while the number of teeth free from decay nearly halved.[29]

Fluoridation is stopped – and teeth get better

In several parts of the world, water fluoridation has been practised and then stopped. What was then expected was that rates of dental caries would start to rise. But to the surprise of dentists, the reverse has happened – teeth have got better.

The town of Kuopio, in eastern Finland, was fluoridated in 1959. Owing to strong opposition by different civic groups, water fluoridation was stopped at the end of 1992. It was a perfect opportunity for Dr L. Seppa and his colleagues of the Institute of Dentistry, University of Oulu, Finland, to examine the claim that this would result in increases in caries. The population of Jyväskylä, whose distribution of demographic and socio-economic characteristics was similar to Kuopio's, acted as the control group. In 1992, 1995 and 1998, independent random samples of all children aged 3, 6, 9, 12 and 15 years were drawn in Kuopio and Jyväskylä. The total numbers of subjects examined were 688, 1,484 and 1,530 in 1992, 1995 and 1998, respectively. Calibrated dentists registered caries clinically and radiographically.

No indication of increasing caries could be found in the previously fluoridated town during the period 1992–98. In both towns, the mean DMFT values either decreased or remained about the same during the observation period.

Some put the decrease down to the use of other fluoridated dental treatments. In fact, the mean numbers of fluoride varnish and sealant applications had also markedly decreased in 1993–98 compared with 1990–92. The conclusion was that teeth got better in Kuopio after fluoridation ceased.[30]

Dr W. Künzel and colleagues at the Dental School of Erfurt, Department of Preventive Dentistry, Friedrich-Schiller-University of Jena, Germany, had similar findings in the former East Germany. In contrast to the anticipated increase in dental caries following the cessation of water fluoridation in the cities of Chemnitz (formerly Karl-Marx-Stadt) and Plauen, a significant fall in caries prevalence was observed. This trend corresponded to the national decline in caries and appeared to be a new population-wide phenomenon. To confirm this 'unexpected epidemiological finding', additional surveys were conducted in the formerly fluoridated towns of Spremberg and Zittau. Pupils from these towns, aged 8–9, 12–13 and 15–16 years, were examined repeatedly over twenty years using standardised procedures. Caries levels for the 12-year-olds of both towns decreased significantly during the years 1993–96, following the cessation of water fluoridation. In Spremberg, DMFT fell by 38.5 per cent, from 2.36 to 1.45, and in Zittau by 20.6 per cent, from 2.47 to 1.96.

Künzel and colleagues say that the mean of 1.81 DMFT for the 12-year-olds, computed from data of the four towns, is the lowest observed in East Germany during the past forty years.[31]

These countries are not in fluoride's heartland. Canada is. After fluoridation ceased in some parts of British Columbia, Dr G. Maupome and fellow researchers at the Faculty of

Dentistry, University of British Columbia, Vancouver, Canada, compared the prevalence and incidence of dental caries in fluoridated and unfluoridated communities in that province. While sources of fluoride other than water fluoridation made it more difficult to detect changes in the epidemiological profile of a population with generally low caries experience, there were measurable differences between the fluoridated and unfluoridated communities.

Maupome and colleagues found that the prevalence of caries *decreased* over time in the community in which fluoridation had ended, while it remained unchanged in the fluoridated community.[32]

Conclusion

Given the strength of the evidence presented, the case for the fluoridation of tap water to prevent dental decay fails miserably. Nevertheless, on both sides of the Atlantic, proponents, seemingly oblivious of this evidence, are currently trying to get still more areas fluoridated. In 1992, when 60 per cent of the US population was drinking fluoridated water, and based on what was described as 'past progress and continuing evidence of effectiveness and safety of this public health measure',[33] the American public health service set a goal of having 75 per cent of the population drinking fluoridated water by the year 2000. And now, as I write this in 2001, the government-funded British Fluoridation Society is actively lobbying for a change in the law to compel water companies to fluoridate tap water in Britain as well.

References

1. Burt BA. Influences for change in the dental health status of populations: an historical perspective. *J Public Health Dent* 1978; 38: 272–88.

2. Klein H. Dental status and dental needs of young adult males, rejectable, or acceptable for military service, according to Selective Service dental requirements. *Public Health Rep* 1941; 56: 1369–87.

3. Dalderup LM. Nutrition and caries. *World Rev Nutr Diet* 1967; 7: 72–137.

4. Davies GN. *Cost and benefit of fluoride in the prevention of dental caries.* Offset Publication, No. 9. World Health Organization, 1974.

5. Martin B. *Scientific knowledge in controversy. The social dynamics of the fluoridation debate.* New York: State University of New York Press, 1991: 16.

6. Foulkes RG. Fluoridation of community water supplies 1992: Update. *Townsend Letter for Doctors* 1992; June: 450. See also *City of Oroville* v. *Public Utilities*, California, 1955, and *Chicago Citizens* v. *City of Chicago*, 1960.

7. *J Am Dent Assoc* 1953; 47: 159–79.

8. *J Am Dent Assoc* 1955; 50: 272–7.

9. Leverett DH. Fluorides and the changing prevalence of dental caries. *Science* 1982; 217: 26–30.

10. World Health Organization. *Oral health global indicator for 2000: Dental caries levels at 12 years.* WHO: Geneva, 1995. See also Hescot P, Roland E. *Dental health in France. DMF scores for 6, 9 and 12 years old.* French Union for Oral Health (UFSBD), 1993.

11. Hileman B. New studies cast doubt on fluoridation benefits. *Chem Eng News* 1989; 67: 5.

12. Gray A. Fluoridation: time for a new baseline? *J Can Dent Assoc* 1987; 10: 272–9.

13. Tijmstra T, Brinkman-Engels M, Groeneveld A. Effect of socioeconomic factors on the observed caries reduction after fluoride tablet and fluoride toothpaste consumption. *Community Dent Oral Epidemiol* 1978; 6: 227–30.

14. Teotia S. Endemic fluoride in bones and teeth – Update. *India J Environ Toxicol* 1991; 1: 1.

15. UK Department of Health. *Fluoridation studies in the United Kingdom and the results achieved after eleven years.* London: HMSO, 1969.

16. Weaver R. The inhibition of dental caries by fluorine. *Proc R Soc Med* 1948; 23 Feb: 284–90.

17. Schatz A. The failure of fluoridation in England. In: *Prevention.* Emmaus, PA: Rodale Press, 1972: 64–9.

18. van Palenstein-Helderman WH, Mabelya L, van't Hof MA, Konig KG. Two types of intraoral distribution of fluorotic enamel. *Community Dent Oral Epidemiol* 1997; 25: 251–5.

19. World Health Organization. *Environmental health criteria. 36: Fluorine and fluorides.* Geneva: WHO, 1984.

20. Murray JJ, Rugg-Gunn AJ. Additional data on water fluoridation. Poster at XXVI ORCA Congress, 1979. Cited in 'WHO: Environmental Health Criteria 36: Fluorine and Fluorides', WHO, Geneva, 1984.

21. Murray JJ, Rugg-Gunn AJ. *Fluorides in caries prevention.* 2nd edn. Wright, Bristol, 1982.

22. Sutton PRN. Fluoridation of water. *Chem Eng News* 1989; 67: 3.

23. Sutton PRN. *Fluoridation: Errors and omissions in experimental trials.* Melbourne: Melbourne University Press, 1959.

24. Gray AS. *J Can Dent Assoc* 1987; 10: 763.

25. Teotia SPS, Teotia M. Dental caries: A disorder of high fluoride and low dietary calcium interactions (30 years of personal research). *Fluoride* 1994; 27: 59–66.

26. Yiamouyiannis J. Water fluoridation and tooth decay: Results from the 1986–1987 national survey of US school children. *Fluoride* 1990; 23: 55–67.

27. Simard PL. Ingestion of fluoride from dentifrices by children aged 12 to 24 months. *Clin Pediatr* 1991; 00:614–17.

28. Imai Y. Relation between fluoride concentration in drinking water and dental caries in Japan. *Koku Eisei Gakkai Zasshi* 1972; 22 (2): 144–96.

29. Scrivener C. Unfavourable report from Kansas community using artificial fluoridation on city water supply for three-year period. *J Dent Res* 1951; 30 (4): 465.

30. Seppa L, Karkkainen S, Hausen H. Caries frequency in permanent teeth before and after discontinuation of water fluoridation in Kuopio, Finland. *Community Dent Oral Epidemiol* 1998; 26: 256–62. See also by same author: Caries in the primary dentition, after discontinuation of water fluoridation, among children receiving comprehensive dental care. *Community Dent Oral Epidemiol* 2000; 28: 281–8.

31. Künzel W, Fischer T, Lorenz R, Bruhmann S. Decline of caries prevalence after the cessation of water fluoridation in the former East Germany. *Community Dent Oral Epidemiol* 2000; 28: 382–9.

32. Maupome G, Clark DC, Levy SM, Berkowitz J. Patterns of dental caries following the cessation of water fluoridation. *Community Dent Oral Epidemiol* 2001; 29: 37–47.

33. US Department of Health and Human Services. *Policy statement on community water fluoridation.* Washington, DC, 22 July 1992.

2. Fluoride and Water Safety

Is fluoridated water safe?

BFS suggested answer

Yes. Every reputable scientific body which has ever considered the issue, including the World Health Organization, the British Medical Association, the British Dental Association and the Health Education Authority, has concluded that water fluoridation is safe.

The World Health Organization recommends that 'water fluoridation is safe and cost-effective and should be introduced and maintained wherever it is socially acceptable and feasible'.

BFS suggested answer refuted

As a toxicologist involved in fluoride research for over ten years, I was stunned by the Calgary Regional Health Authority's glib comments proclaiming water fluoridation safe. The 'fifty years' of studies about fluoride safety do not exist. The 'ongoing intensive research on fluorides and fluoridation' does not exist, certainly none investigating safety.
Professor Phyllis Mullenix, 1997

This question, like the previous one, is fundamental to fluoridation. Even if adding fluoride to drinking water did benefit teeth, those who advocate it would, clearly, have to reconsider its addition if it were shown that in benefitting some, they harmed others.

Calcium fluoride (CaF)

The fluoride which occurs naturally in drinking water all over the world is calcium fluoride (i.e. fluorine + calcium), or

33

sometimes magnesium fluoride (fluorine + magnesium). In Britain, calcium fluoride is usually found at low levels of around 0.01–0.1 ppm. At these low levels, calcium fluoride is relatively insoluble and passes relatively harmlessly through the body. Nevertheless, calcium fluoride can accumulate in bone, teeth and other body tissues. In some areas of the world, calcium fluoride levels are of great public health concern. In sixteen states in India, for example, with calcium fluoride levels between 5 and 13 ppm, chronic skeletal fluorosis is endemic, and 6 million children are so crippled that they cannot walk to school. Although that is not the situation in Europe, dental fluorosis, acknowledged by Baroness Hayman to be a sign of systemic toxicity, has been observed and documented at levels in water as low as 0.34 ppm.[1] That is only one-third the amount recommended for water fluoridation here.

The original studies of fluoridation were done in areas with 'high' (up to 1 ppm) levels of naturally occurring calcium fluoride. But calcium fluoride has never been used for artificial fluoridation of drinking water.

Sodium fluoride (NaF)

All clinical laboratory testing of fluoride has been conducted using rats as the subjects – despite the fact that rats rarely suffer from tooth decay. As contaminated materials could compromise the results of the trials, animal trials were conducted using a pharmaceutical grade of sodium fluoride (fluorine + sodium), with purified water and high-grade feed. When the rats did not develop tooth decay (although they did develop dental fluorosis), it was said that this is proof that 'fluoride reduces tooth decay'. This pure grade of sodium fluoride is 'deemed' to be a suitable surrogate for naturally occurring calcium fluoride. It is also 'deemed' to be a suitable surrogate for water artificially fluoridated with hexafluorosilicic acid (H_2SiF_6).

Sodium fluoride is not used for the artificial fluoridation of drinking water in Britain or Ireland, but it is used in toothpastes and other fluoridated dental preparations.

Fluorosilicates

The only 'fluorides' that the law in Britain and Ireland allows to be used for water fluoridation are the fluorosilicates, hexafluorosilicic acid (H_2SiF_6) and its sodium salt, disodium hexafluorosilicate (Na_2SiF_6).[2] These 'fluorosilicates', as their name implies, contain silicon, but it is not listed. This omission is significant, because if it were listed, it would *have* to be labelled and subjected to toxicological studies, as silicon is known to cause cancer. If that weren't bad enough, these fluorosilicates, in the form in which they are added to drinking water, are not pure. As will be discussed in Chapter 25, they are classified as 'hazardous air pollutants'.

In order to minimise emissions to air of hazardous air pollutants, the gases produced in the phosphate fertiliser manufacturing process are 'washed' in 'pollution scrubbers', and the resulting 'gravy', as it is called, is collected for disposal or sale. As such, the product is not a pure chemical. Approximately 19 per cent is fluorine; the rest is a toxic soup containing lead, arsenic, beryllium, vanadium, cadmium, mercury, radionuclides and, of course, silicon.

The presence of these contaminants is of great concern. Arsenic is classified as a Group 1 known human carcinogen; beryllium is also classified as a known human carcinogen; lead is a known neurotoxicant; arsenic, lead and fluoride are cumulative toxins.

Chromium is another known carcinogen. John Gormley, TD, asked the Irish Minister for Health whether chromium was present in the hydrofluorosilicic acid imported from Holland to fluoridate Irish drinking water. The Minister said categorically that it was not. However, the Irish organisation

Fluoride Free Water had an independent chemical analysis done on the chemical cocktail. It showed that chromium levels were 3.763 ppm and that levels of arsenic were even higher at 4.829 ppm. On 7 November 2000, the Minister apologised for misleading the Dáil.[3] 'According to the Irish Medicines Board, this hydrofluosilicic [hydrofluorosilicic] acid has never been proven safe or effective', said dental surgeon Dr Don MacAuley. 'Not surprisingly it is unregistered, unlicensed and not considered to be a medicine.'[4]

Conclusion

No safety tests have ever been done on silicofluorides. There are no proper studies on the effectiveness of hexafluorosilicic acid in reducing dental caries either. Many of the components of the 'product' that is used for water fluoridation are known to be extremely harmful, yet no safety testing data are available for it anywhere in the world.

Any claim that 'water fluoridation is safe' is at best wishful thinking and at worst a lie.

References

1. Lin F-F, Aihaiti, Zhao HX et al. The relationship of a low-iodine and high-fluoride environment to subclinical cretinism in Xinjiang. *IDD Newsletter* vol. 7, no. 3, August 1991.

2. Water (Fluoridation) Act, Chapter 63. London: HMSO, 1985: 1–4.

3. Written answer to Dáil question no. 598, 7 November 2000.

4. Troubled water: Minister accused of lying over tap water chemicals. *Evening Herald* (Ireland), 8 September 2000.

3. Cancer and Fluoride

Is it true that young males living in fluoridated communities have an increased risk of bone cancer?

BFS suggested answer

No. The evidence on fluoridation and cancer – including bone cancer – has been reviewed by expert committees – including the Knox committee here in the UK, and the National Cancer Institute in the USA. There is no evidence whatsoever to support the claim that fluoridated water is associated with an increase in cancer anywhere in the body.

BFS suggested answer refuted

The mutagenicity of fluoride supports the conclusion that fluoride is a probable human carcinogen. An important toxicologic consideration is that a toxic substance stores at the same place it exerts its toxic activity.
Dr William Marcus, Environmental Protection Agency scientist

Fluoride and genetic damage

Many studies have noted a link between fluoride and genetic toxicity. Dr W. Klein and colleagues at Austria's Siebersdorf Research Centre found in 1977 that 1 ppm fluoride inhibited DNA repair enzyme activity by 50 per cent and caused genetic and chromosome damage.[1] This was confirmed in 1982 at the University of Missouri.[2] Sperm cells were damaged by fluoride in a test carried out at Holland's Leiden University, leading to a 'highly significant increase in mutation'.[3]

Scientists at the West German Central Laboratory for Mutagenicity Testing[4] and at Columbia University[5] came up with similar findings showing that fluoride also caused genetic damage to eggs in both insects and mammals. And a committee of the National Research Council of Canada, which reviewed the research in 1977, concluded that 'fluoride has displayed mutagenic activity in studies of vegetation, insects, and mammalian oocytes. There is a high correlation between carcinogenicity and mutagenicity of pollutants, and fluoride has been one of the major pollutants in several situations where a high incidence of respiratory cancer has been observed.'

In 1993 the US National Institutes of Environmental Health Sciences stated: 'In cultured human and rodent cells, the weight of evidence leads to the conclusion that fluoride exposure results in increased chromosome aberrations.'[6]

In Poland, scientists at the Pomeranian Medical Academy reported that as little as 0.6 ppm fluoride produced chromosomal damage to human white blood cells.[7]

Even Procter & Gamble, which makes Crest (fluoridated) toothpaste, produced a study showing that 1 ppm fluoride causes genetic damage[8] – so it's no secret.

Fluoride and cancer

A mutagen is a substance that can induce genetic mutations in an organism: changes that may affect the structure, development and physical characteristics of any subsequent offspring. Similarly, a carcinogen is a substance that can cause cancer. The two may be very similar, and many substances that cause mutations also cause cancer. Scientists in several countries have demonstrated that this is the case with fluoride.

Dr R.A. Holman of the Royal Institute of Pathology stated in 1961:

> Fluoride is a well-known inhibitor of several enzyme systems, and can form spectroscopically recognizable compounds with the enzyme *catalase*, resulting in its

inhibition. Catalase poisoning has been linked with the development of viruses and the causation of several diseases, including cancer. Many observers have suggested that the agents (fluorides and other toxic environmental substances) which decrease the catalase in the cells may predispose those cells to tumour formation.[9]

In the USA, a comparison between the ten largest fluoridated cities and the ten largest unfluoridated cities showed that, whereas cancer rates had been similar initially, after twenty years the fluoridated cities had 10 per cent more cancer deaths than the unfluoridated ones.[10] These figures were checked and confirmed in 1976 by the US National Cancer Institute.

The 1987 figures for the incidence of registered cancers in communities in the USA and the 1985 fluoridation census by the US Department of Health and Human Services enabled scientists to conduct an epidemiological analysis of the correlation between the two in the United States. They found significant correlations in both sexes between water fluoridation and numbers of cancers of the digestive system (tongue, mouth, pharynx, oesophagus, stomach, colon, rectum and pancreas), the respiratory system (larynx, bronchi and lungs), and the renal system. In the sexual organs, contradictions were seen. In women, cancers of the breast, cervix and ovary were increased in fluoridated areas, whereas in males those of the prostate, testis and penis were apparently inhibited. The authors considered that the different effects suggest that fluoride may act as an environmental hormone. The dose–response relationship between the numbers of bone cancers in male teenagers and the amount of fluoridation was statistically significant. These significant relationships indicated that fluoride may be, not an initiator, but a promoter of cancer.[11]

The world's leading authority on the biological effects of fluoride, Dr John Yiamouyiannis, estimates that 30,000–50,000 deaths each year in the United States are directly attributable to fluoride.[12] Dr Dean Burk, the chief chemist emeritus of the US National Cancer Institute, agreed. 'In point of fact, fluoride causes more human cancer death, and causes it faster, than any other chemical', he said.

The cancer link is covered up

Osteosarcoma is a rare form of bone cancer, but it is the most common form of bone cancer in children and one of the principal cancers of childhood.

Because of concerns that fluoride might cause cancer, in 1977 the US Congress ordered the US Department of Health and Human Services to conduct the National Toxicology Program animal study. The results were published in 1990.[13] The study showed that sodium fluoride caused osteosclerosis (abnormal bone density), oral tumours, a rare bone cancer (osteosarcoma) and a rare liver cancer called hepato-cholangiocarcinoma at cumulative dosages comparable to those ingested by humans over a number of years.

Normally, when a drug is being tested, two groups of people or animals are selected to be as nearly alike as possible. One, the *intervention group*, has the drug, while the other, called the *control group*, has none. After a period of time, the two groups are compared and any differences detected. But this did not happen in the NTP study: the control group also received fluoride, albeit at a lower rate.[14] Thus, the control animals were not controls at all, but low-dosage experimental animals. This raised the level of cancers observed in all animals and hid the effect supposedly being studied, leading to a finding that fluoride did not cause cancer.

Drs Robert Carton and William Marcus noted this and a number of other problems, including the fact that many of the cancers found were downgraded to commoner types, which had the effect of downgrading the results still further, or even eliminating them altogether.[15] Despite these manipulations, the occurrence of osteosarcoma, an unusual cancer for rodents, in male rats showed a statistically significant positive linear relationship to fluoride dosage. In other words, the more fluoride the rodents had, the more cancers they developed.

On 26 April 1990, a conference was held to peer-review the NTP draft report. Dr Marcus, senior science advisor, Criteria and Standards Division, wrote a memo to its acting director, Alan B. Hais, reporting that he was disturbed by much of what he read in the NTP report:

> The highest dosed level of rats had lower levels of fluoride in their bones (5,470 ppm) compared to people (7,000 ppm) at the MCL [maximum contaminant level] of 4 ppm. This can be interpreted as people who ingest drinking water at the MCL have 1.3 times more fluoride in their bones than male rats who get osteosarcoma. This is the first time in my memory that animals have lower concentrations of the carcinogen at the site of adverse effect than do humans. An important toxicologic consideration is that a toxic substance stores at the same place it exerts its toxic activity. This is true of benzene and now for fluoride. Fluoride, however, is at twice the concentration in human bones compared to benzene, which is 10 to 100 [times] greater in animal marrow. This portends a very serious problem.[16]

The fluoride dosages in this study were comparatively low: the doses of other substances tested for carcinogenicity ranged from 6 to 500 times the fluoride dosage (see Table 1). This study is highly relevant, as the average cumulative dosage of fluoride ingested by people living in fluoridated communities reaches that of the low-dosage rats after only thirty-eight years; for many people, the average cumulative dosage will equal that of the mid-dosage rats in a lifetime, and for some will even approach that of the high-dosage rats.

Substance	Daily dose (mg/kg)	MCL (mg/litre)
Fluoride	7.9[a]	4
Carbon tetrachloride	47	0.005
Benzene	50	0.005
Chloroform	160	0.1
Tetrachloroethylene	386	0.005
Red dye #3	4000	None

Source: Professor David R. Hill, *Fluoride: Risks and Benefits. Disinformation in the service of big industry.* Presented in Calgary's Operation and Environment Committee, 10 September 1997.

[a]This fluoride dosage caused bone cancer in male rats.

Table 1. Comparison of dosages used to test suspected carcinogens, and the maximum contaminant levels (MCL) allowed

Despite all the machinations, the NTP study did not give fluoride a clean bill of health. Fluoride's particular affinity for bone adds to the significance of the link with the bone cancers that affected males.

Animal trials are confirmed in human studies

In the light of the NTP study on rodents and of epidemiologic evidence of an increase in a bone cancer, osteosarcoma, in boys and young men, especially in fluoridated areas, Dr Perry Cohn of the New Jersey Department of Health in America surveyed the incidence of this cancer in seven counties of New Jersey relative to water fluoridation. He found that, as demonstrated in Table 2, the incidence of osteosarcoma in boys in the fluoridated areas was up to 4.6 times higher than in the unfluoridated areas.[17] In a similar study of three New Jersey municipalities, the incidence of osteosarcoma reached levels nearly seven times higher in the fluoridated than in the unfluoridated areas. Cohn also found that the general population in the fluoridated areas was five times as likely to suffer from cancer.

Age	Area fluoridation status	No. of cases	Population	Rates of osteosarcoma[a]
	Seven counties, New Jersey, USA, 1979–87			
0–9	Fluoridated	2	48,129	4.6
	Unfluoridated	1	102,123	1.0
10–19	Fluoridated	10	62,990	17.6
	Unfluoridated	7	151,384	5.1
20–49	Fluoridated	5	141,429	3.9
	Unfluoridated	5	348,570	1.5
	Three municipalities, New Jersey, USA, 1979–87			
0–9	Fluoridated	2	38,654	5.7
	Unfluoridated	1	46,708	2.3
10–19	Fluoridated	10	50,297	20.0
	Unfluoridated	2	67,678	3.2
20–49	Fluoridated	4	115,367	3.8
	Unfluoridated	2	153,713	1.4

Source: Cohn PD. *A brief report on the association of drinking water fluoridation and the incidence of osteosarcoma among young males.* Trenton, NJ: New Jersey Department of Health, 8 November 1992.

[a]Per 100,000.

Table 2. Fluoride and osteosarcoma in young males

It is not surprising that any cancer caused by fluoride should be a bone cancer, and it is equally unsurprising that it should occur in the young, as fluoride accumulates primarily in bones, and children, who are actively forming bone, have a higher uptake of fluoride into bone than adults. Further, bone in knees, ankles, shoulders and wrists, where childhood osteosarcoma most often occurs, shows a high response to fluoride.[18]

Cohn's study also showed that fluoride affects males differently from females – whereas male cancers tended to be of the bones, females were more susceptible to soft-tissue cancers. This means it is important to consider the sexes separately in trials to avoid watering down, and thus hiding, significant effects. This has not been done.

Given the large number of people in the New Jersey study, and given the results of the NTP study, you might expect alarm bells to have rung loudly for the US public health system, especially as the US Department of Health and Human Services had previously noted a rise in such cancers among young males in fluoridated areas during the first five years of fluoridation.[19] Instead, the executive summary of the NTP, which is the only part likely to be read by high-ranking government officials, starts by praising the dental benefits of fluoridation, and then fails to present the results clearly.

Many people in Britain and Ireland ingest more than the 'optimum' amount of fluoride, some by six times or more.[20] With increasingly widespread fluoride contamination, these amounts will rise, in which case it will take less time to accumulate dosages similar to those of the rats.

Other cancers

Fluoride may have a causal relationship with more than just bone cancer in males:

Respiratory cancer

An environmental committee of Canada's National Research Council stated in 1977: 'Fluoride is a persistent bioaccumulator . . . There is a high correlation between carcinogenicity and mutagenicity of pollutants, and **fluoride has been one of the major pollutants in several situations where a high incidence of respiratory cancer has been observed.**'[21] (Emphasis added)

Oral cancer

The NTP rat study also noted an increase in oral cancers in the rat. Combined oral papilloma and carcinoma approached statistical significance in males in the trend test. The NTP did not consider these tumours to be related to fluoride intakes and concluded that the finding pointed to a possible, but not yet probable, relationship. However, oral cancer rates in humans have risen markedly in the last few decades, despite the fact that smoking is on the decrease.

Uterine cancer

The Japanese Ryukyu Islands, including the island of Okinawa, were under US administration from 1945 to 1972. During that time, fluoride was added to the drinking water in most regions. It was a unique opportunity to study the effects of the change. Dr E. Tohyama of the Department of Preventive Medicine, School of Medicine, University of the Ryukyus, Okinawa, studied the relationship between fluoride concentration in drinking water and uterine cancer death rates in twenty Okinawan towns over the period.[22] The study results were noteworthy:

- A significant positive correlation existed between fluoride concentration in drinking water and uterine cancer deaths.

- This association remained significant even after adjusting for the potential confounding variables.

- The time trends in the uterine cancer deaths were related to changes in water fluoridation practices.

Tohyama wasn't the first Japanese to look for links between fluoride and cancer. Researchers there had achieved a degree of understanding of fluoride consumption and human cancer by 1984. Using levels of fluoride that, according to the US National Cancer Institute, would determine whether fluoridation of public drinking water caused cancer, Dr Takeki Tsutsui of the Nippon Dental College showed that 'fluoride caused not only genetic damage but was also capable of transforming normal human cells into cancer cells'.[23]

Tsutsui's work in Japan was confirmed in 1988 by researchers at the Argonne National Laboratory in France.[24] They also discovered that fluoride has a synergistic effect with other cancer-causing chemicals in the food and environment. Interestingly, this work confirmed yet more studies sponsored by the US National Cancer Institute. In 1963, low levels of fluoride increased the rate of melanomas in living organisms from 12 to 100 per cent in a study at University of Missouri, Saint Louis.[25] These studies were further amplified by work done at the University of Texas by the Taylors, who found that 1 ppm fluoride in drinking water increased tumour growth rate in mice by 25 per cent.[26] Fluoride, like mercury and lead, suppressed the immune system.

According to Dr John Yiamouyiannis, studies in the United States and Canada have shown that cancer death rates are from 4 to 40 per cent higher in areas where the water is fluoridated than in areas where it is not.

Conclusion

This is a small taste of the vast amount of literature detailing fluoride's ability to cause genetic and chromosomal damage to body cells. All cancers are, after all, caused merely by changes to a cell's DNA.

The American Food and Drug Administration (FDA) does not allow anything that has been shown to be carcinogenic in animal tests to be put in food. Even if fluoride did not cause cancer in humans, the fact that it does so in animals should automatically bar it from entering the food chain.

References

1. Klein W et al. DNA repair and environmental substances. *Z Angew Bader- Klimaheilkunde* 1977; 24 (3): 218–23.

2. Mohamed A, Chandler ME. Cytological effects of sodium fluoride on mice. *Fluoride* 1982; 15 (3): 110–18.

3. Mukerjee RN, Sobels FH. The effect of sodium fluoride and iodoacetamide on mutation induction by X-irradiation in mature spermatozoa of *Drosophila*. *Mutat Res* 1968; 6: 217–25.

4. Vogel E. Strong antimutagenic effects of fluoride on mutation induction by trenimon and 1-phenyl-3,3-dimethyltriazine in *Drosophila melanogaster*. *Mutat Res* 1973; 20: 339–52.

5. Jagiello G, Lin J-S. Sodium fluoride as potential mutagen in mammalian eggs. *Arch Environ Health* 1974; 29: 230–5.

6. Zeiger E, Shelby MD, Witt KL. Genetic toxicity of fluoride. *Environ Mol Mutagen* 1993; 21: 309–18.

7. Jachimczak D, Skotarczak B. The effect of fluorine and lead ions on the chromosomes of human leucocytes in vitro. *Genet Pol* 1978; 19 (3): 353–7.

8. Aarderna MJ, Gibson DP, Leboeuf RA. Sodium fluoride-induced chromosome aberrations in different stages of the cell cycle: a proposed mechanism. *Mutat Res* 1989; 223: 191–203.

9. Holman RA. Prevention of dental caries. *Br Med J* 1961; 1110–11.

10. Yiamouyiannis JA, Burk D. Fluoridation of public water systems and the cancer death rate in humans. Presented at the 67th Annual Meeting of the American Society of Biologists and Chemists and the American Society of Experimental Biologists, June 1976.

11. Takahashi K, Akiniwa K, Narita K. Cancer-promoting power of fluoridation. Presented at the 22nd Conference of the International Society for Fluoride Research, Bellingham, Washington, USA, 24–27 August 1998.

12. Yiamouyiannis JA. *Fluoride: The aging factor*. Delaware, OH: Health Action Press, 1983.

13. *Toxicology and carcinogenesis studies of sodium fluoride (CAS No. 7681-49-4) in F344/N rats and B6C3F1 mice.* National Toxicology Program Technical Report TR 393. National Institutes of Health, US Department of Health and Human Services, 1990.

14. US Department of Health and Human Services Subcommittee Review, 1991: 73.

15. Carton RJ, Marcus WL. Internal memorandums from the US Environmental Protection Agency, where Dr Carton was an environmental scientist and Dr Marcus a senior science advisor and toxicologist in the Office of Drinking Water. The memorandums are dated 1 May 1990, 1 June 1990, 24 September 1990 and 18 October 1990.

16. Marcus WL. Fluoride conference to review the NTP draft fluoride report. Memorandum to Alan B. Hais. US Environmental Protection Agency, 1 May 1990.

17. Cohn PD. *A brief report on the association of drinking water fluoridation and the incidence of osteosarcoma among young males.* Trenton, New Jersey: New Jersey Department of Health, 8 November 1992.

18. Gelberg KH, Fitzgerald EF, Hwang S, Dubrow R. Fluoride exposure and childhood osteosarcoma: A case control study. *Am J Public Health* 1995; 85: 1678–83.

19. US Department of Health and Human Services Subcommittee Review, 1991: 82.

20. Mansfield P. *We underestimate the damage done by fluorides.* Mansfield, Louth, Lincs, 1997.

21. Associate Committee On Scientific Criteria For Environmental Quality. *Environmental fluoride.* NRCC No. 16081. National Research Council of Canada, 1977.

22. Tohyama E. Relationship between fluoride concentration in drinking water and mortality rate from uterine cancer in Okinawa prefecture, Japan. *J Epidemiol* 1996; 6: 184–91.

23. Tsutsui T, Suzuki N, Ohmori M. Sodium fluoride induced morphological and neoplastic transformation, chromosome aberrations, sister chromatid exchanges and unscheduled DNA synthesis in cultured Syrian hamster embryo cells. *Cancer Res* 1984; 44: 938–41.
24. Jones CA, Callahan MF, Huberman E. Sodium fluoride promotes morphological transformation of Syrian hamster embryo cells. *Carcinogenesis* 1988; 9: 2279–84.
25. Herskowitz IH, Norton IL. Increased incidence of melanotic tumors in two strains of *Drosophila melanogaster* following treatment with sodium fluoride. *Genetics* 1963; 48: 307–10.
26. Taylor A, Taylor NC. Effect of sodium fluoride on tumor growth. *Proc Soc Exp Biol Med* 1965; 119: 252–5.

4. Safe Limit for Fluoride

The National Pure Water Association says we are already ingesting more than the government's safe limit. Do you agree?

BFS suggested answer
No. There is no evidence to support that claim. The so-called safe limit quoted by NPWA does not exist.

This claim is a misrepresentation of the term 'safe intake' as it is used in a Department of Health report. The report explains that 'safe intakes' are not intended as a 'toxic level'. In fact it states that there is a wide safety margin above the more usual intakes in fluoridated areas. This has been pointed out to the NPWA on several occasions.

BFS suggested answer refuted
The most important and widely disregarded fact about dental fluorosis is that no safe established daily intake exists, i.e., the maximal amount in mg fluoride which, consumed daily, does not produce cosmetically damaging white areas or brown stain in some areas has not been fixed.
Dr Harold C. Hodge

The proponents of fluoridation have always insisted that fluoride has no adverse side effects: that it is quite harmless, that it does nothing other than strengthen teeth. Throughout this book you will see evidence which shows that much of that statement is suspect. The first suspicion that this is so comes in declarations by health authorities that fluoridated drinking water is perfectly safe[1] – followed by recommendations for a safe or a maximum limit for daily intake.

The currently recommended level of 1 ppm (part per million) fluoride in drinking water aims to provide for a total intake of 1 mg per day. This assumes that an individual drinks 1 litre of water per day, despite the fact that health experts recommend an intake of three times that amount and even more in hot weather.

The bodge by Hodge

It is important when any new drug is marketed that the exposure at which it is toxic is determined. Then a margin is allowed for safety (usually a factor of 100) and a maximum exposure published.

In 1953 the National Academy of Sciences published their estimate of the quantity of fluoride which produces the condition known as crippling skeletal fluorosis. The calculation was done by a famous toxicologist, Harold C. Hodge, PhD, who at that time was chairman of the US National Academy of Sciences (NAS) committee on toxicology.

To arrive at his figures, Hodge cited the classic study of the effects of fluoride among cryolite workers published in 1937 by European researcher, Kaj Roholm.[2] Roholm's dosage figures, presented in milligrams of fluoride per kilogram of body weight, showed that at levels of 0.2–0.35 mg/kg, the first stage of the disease appeared, in general, after two and a half years; stage 2 was reached by four and a half years; and crippling skeletal fluorosis appeared after eleven years.

Hodge wanted to apply Roholm's figures to a typical range of body weights in order to set a maximum intake level in milligrams per day. But Hodge, an American, was used to dealing in pounds rather than kilograms. Using body weights from 100 to 229 pounds, he multiplied the 0.2 mg figure by 100 pounds, giving a figure of 20 mg/day; and 0.35 mg by 229 pounds to give 80 mg/day. Thus, the amounts of fluoride that would cause crippling skeletal fluorosis, he said, were 20–80 mg/day for a period of ten to twenty years. These are the figures that appear in the American Dental Association's pamphlet, *Fluoridation Facts*, and on which many other articles are based, even today.

But Hodge had made a simple but significant error: in converting fluoride amounts from milligrams per kilogram to milligrams per pound, he got it wrong. Unfortunately, Hodge was the expert, and no-one, apparently, queried or even checked his figures. This error, which gave a false safety margin more than double what it should have been, went unnoticed for many years until an American anti-fluoride campaigner, Darlene Sherrell, tried to duplicate Hodge's arithmetic and couldn't make the figures add up.

Correcting for the error, Sherrell reduced the amount of fluoride needed to be crippling to 10–25 mg/day, over a period of ten to twenty years. Duration of exposure is important, because fluorides accumulate in our bodies throughout our lives, so a higher intake over a shorter period of time will have the same effect as smaller doses over a longer period of time. If we apply Roholm's dosage figures to a lifetime of 55–96 years, just 1 mg per day (the amount in 1 litre of water) for each 55 pounds of body weight could be a crippling dosage.

The NAS admits it was wrong

In 1979 Hodge corrected his previous figures in a book, *Continuing Evaluation of the Use of Fluorides*, but nobody seems to have noticed. Sherrell wrote to the National Academy of Sciences in 1989. In 1991, when scientists at the US Department of Health and Human Services published their *Review of Fluoride: Benefits and Risks*, they continued to use figures of 20–80 mg/day as the 'crippling daily dose of fluoride'. The error was finally corrected by the National Research Council's Board on Environmental Studies and Toxicology in 1993, when they changed the figure from

20–80 mg/day to 10–20 mg/day.[3] Even today, the current recommended daily allowance (RDA) and dietary reference intakes, published by the US Institute of Medicine, still use the wrong figures.

Myths are very hard to dislodge.

'Optimum' levels and safe limits

When 1 ppm fluoride was first recommended, water was about the only source of fluoride in diet. Today that is no longer the case. Studies indicate that total fluoride ingestion today approaches 4.0 mg per day *even in areas without water fluoridation*. Commercial beverages may be manufactured with fluoridated water; it is present in foods; toothpastes and oral hygiene products contain substantial amounts of fluoride, as do some medications. Thus, even in unfluoridated areas, many now receive substantially more fluoride than the 'ideal' amount.

In 1996, for the first time, the UK Department of Health published safe fluoride intakes at various ages: in adults, the Department of Health suggests that this is 3 mg per day.[4] This differs from the American standard, and this flat rate also takes no account of differences in age, size, ambient temperature – we drink more when we are hot – or any other factor. The USA's Nutrition Board of the Institute of Medicine attempted to address this problem, basing intakes on age and body weight (see Table 1).

But no matter what scales are used, just how meaningful are safe intakes? People drink different amounts of water each day. At an 'optimal' concentration of 1 ppm, the British 3 mg/day is the amount found in just 3 litres, or 5 pints, of water. Tea, grown in areas with high concentrations of fluorine in the soil, is itself a significant source of fluoride in Britain and Ireland.

Age group	Reference weights		Adequate intake (mg/day)	Tolerable upper intake (mg/day)
	kg	(lb)[a]		
Infants 0–6 months	7	(16)	0.01	0.7
Infants 6–12 months	9	(20)	0.5	0.9
Children 1–3 years	13	(29)	0.7	1.3
Children 4–8 years	22	(48)	1.0	2.0
Children 9–13 years	40	(88)	2.0	10
Boys 14–18 years	64	(142)	3.0	10
Girls 14–18 years	57	(125)	3.0	10
Females 19+ years	76	(166)	4.0	10
Males 19+ years	61	(133)	3.0	10

[a]Values based on data collected between 1988 and 1994 as part of the Third Health and Nutrition Examination Survey (NHANES III) in the United States.

Table 1. *Dietary reference intakes for fluoride*

In 1953 it was reckoned that 'exclusive of drinking water, the average diet in the United States is calculated to provide 0.2 to 0.3 milligrams of fluoride daily. Drinking water . . . can provide an optimal internal supplement of approximately one-half to 1 milligram of fluoride per day.'[5] In 1974, average intake was from about 1.7 to 3.44 mg/day. Three years later, the dangers of such a high level of intake were revealed by the National Academy of Sciences:

> Recent studies indicate that the total intake of fluoride is as high as 3 mg/day rather than the earlier figure of 1.5 mg/day, primarily because of increases in the estimated levels of fluoride in food. Balance data presented by Spencer also suggest a higher retention by bone, nearly 2 mg/day, rather than the 0.2 mg/day indicated earlier . . . These findings are important . . . a retention of 2 mg/day would mean that an average individual would experience skeletal fluorosis after 40 yrs.[6]

Despite such warnings, by 1991, the average fluoride intake in fluoridated American cities had more than doubled to over 6.5 mg daily.[7] Current intake is now approaching 8 mg per day, not just from tap water, but from toothpaste and other dental products, beverages, processed foods, fresh fruits and vegetables, pharmaceuticals, Teflon- and Tefal-coated cookware, vitamins and mineral supplements, tea, air . . . the list is endless. This relentless increase in fluorides in our diet means that '[i]t is no longer feasible to estimate with reasonable accuracy the level of fluoride exposure simply on the basis of concentration in drinking water supply'.[8]

It's worse for children

Scientists at the Dental Research Unit, Wellington School of Medicine, New Zealand, analysed 532 juices and juice drinks for fluoride and found concentrations that ranged as high as 2.80 ppm, in part because of the fluoride in water used in production. They say that children's ingestion of fluoride from juices and juice-flavoured drinks can be a substantial factor in the development of fluorosis.[9] A study of 332 fizzy drinks had similar findings in 1999.[10]

Sales of bottled drinking waters in the United Kingdom tripled between 1989 and 1994. Analysis of the fluoride content of twelve bottled waters purchased in 1994 from two Leeds supermarkets showed that they contained from 0.10 to 0.80 ppm fluoride.[11] Although the bottles' labels listed fluoride concentrations, most were inaccurate. The authors of this study warn that some parents using bottled waters to prepare baby milk formulations that themselves may contain high levels of fluoride may subject their children to the risk of dental fluorosis. Dr S. Levy and colleagues of Iowa City confirmed this the following year. They found that water fluoride intake in infants up to nine months old from reconstituted concentrated infant formula ranged as high as

1.57 mg per day.[12] This is up to 157 times the adequate intake and more than double the tolerable upper intake for infants of this age, as defined by the US Third National Health and Nutrition Examination Survey, NHANES III.

The pesticide cryolite, which is 54.3 per cent fluorine, is found on apples, raisins, lettuce, tomatoes, potatoes, peaches, and most berries.[13] The American Consumers Union stated that just one serving of some popular fruits and vegetables could contain enough harmful chemicals to exceed US government health standards – not surprising when almost half of forty-three ready-to-drink fruit juices contained more than 1.0 ppm fluoride, with grape juice containing up to 6.8 ppm.[14] The ACU concluded that children were most at risk – in part because their bodies are more sensitive, but also because they typically consume more fresh fruit for their weight than adults.[15]

The *Journal of the Canadian Dental Association* states: 'Fluoride supplements should not be recommended for children less than 3 years old.'[16] Also: 'The ADA recommends the use of fluoride mouth rinses, but not for children under six years of age because they may swallow the rinse.'[17] If fluoride really is safe, why does swallowing it matter?

In 1995 the *Journal of the American Dental Association* (*JADA*) proclaimed:

> Some children had estimated fluoride intake from water, supplements and dentifrice that exceeded the recommended 'optimal' intake (**a level that has yet to be determined scientifically**). Practitioners should estimate fluoride ingestion from all of these sources if considering systematic fluoride supplementation.[18] [emphasis added]

But wait – a level that has yet to be determined scientifically? What kind of people will recommend giving a medication to the whole population, while admitting that after more than fifty years of so doing, they still haven't determined what the 'optimal' level is?

And that question prompts still more questions:

- If we haven't determined what the 'optimal' level is, how meaningful is it to publish one?

- More importantly, what evidence is there that this level is both effective and safe?

- And how are different people, with different lifestyles, to be protected from ingesting too much? Different people consume different amounts of fluoridated water. For example, athletes, labourers, diabetics and residents of hot or dry regions may drink more water, and therefore more fluoride, than do other people.[19] As a result, it is impossible accurately to control the dosage of fluoride any person ingests.

A safe level should be defined

Before addition to foods, all chemical additives have to be tested for toxicity. After determination of the amount found to be toxic 'to the average person', this amount is divided again to ensure that the amount 'will be safe for almost everybody'. For some unaccountable reason, this is not the case with fluoride. The level of fluoride that is deemed 'optimal' is separated by only a small amount from the amounts that are known to be harmful. Dr James Patrick, a former antibiotics research scientist at the US National Institutes of Health, described this fine distinction:

> [There is] a very low margin of safety involved in fluoridating water. A concentration of about 1 ppm is recommended . . . in several countries, severe fluorosis has been documented from water supplies containing only 2 or 3 ppm. In the development of drugs . . . we generally insist on a therapeutic index [margin of safety] of the order of 100; a therapeutic index of 2 or 3 is

> totally unacceptable, yet that is what has been proposed
> for public water supplies.[20]

In other words, if the rules for other chemicals were applied to
a chemical as ubiquitous as calcium fluoride, the only safe level
in an essential public resource such as drinking water would be
no more than 0.01 ppm. Given this parameter, should we not
now be pursuing a very strict policy of *removing* as much
calcium fluoride as possible from what we eat and drink?
There should certainly be no suggestion of adding any.

Conclusion

The answer that the BFS suggests is strictly correct. But it is a
cleverly worded question and answer. There is no such thing
as a British government safe *limit* for the simple reason that
no government body has ever bothered to determine just how
much fluoride is safe. There is, however, a British safe *intake*:
it is 3 mg per day for an adult. You may wonder what is the
significance of publishing a safe intake, if it is not related to
an *unsafe* intake?

We know from Roholm's figures that an intake of 3 mg
per day has the potential to cause crippling skeletal fluorosis
well within a normal lifetime. Thus, there is certainly *not*
'a wide safety margin above the more usual intakes in
fluoridated areas'.

It is impossible for members of the public to determine
how much fluoride they are ingesting. Even if you avoid
commercially packaged foods and drinks, as I do, there is a
plentiful supply of fluoride in fresh foods, as food animals
may drink fluoridated water, while crops are sprayed with
fluoride-based (cryolite) pesticides and, when picked, may be
washed or packed in fluoridated water.

Incidentally, the city of Natick, Massachusetts, USA, was
forced to fluoridate its water supplies by the public health
service in 1998. Natick selectmen, the town's top elected

officials, are responsible for warning residents any time they are in danger. Following fluoridation, water bills sent to all users carried the following warning printed in bold letters:

> **This water contains fluoride per order of the Natick Board of Health.**
>
> **We recommend that pregnant women, parents of children under 3 years of age, and individuals with known fluoride sensitivity consult with their personal physicians before drinking this water.**[21]

That's how safe they think fluoridated drinking water is!

References

1. Scarrott D. British Dental Association. Personal correspondence to author. 5 June 1997.
2. Roholm K. *Fluorine intoxication. A clinical–hygienic study.* Copenhagen: Nyt Nordisk, and London: HK Lewis, 1937: 281–2.
3. *Health effects of ingested fluoride.* US National Academy of Sciences, 1993: 59.
4. UK Department of Health. *Report on health and social subjects. 41: Dietary reference values for food energy and nutrients for the United Kingdom.* 8th impression. London: HMSO, 1996: 189.
5. *The problem of providing optimum fluoride intake for prevention of dental caries.* Food and Nutrition Board, Division of Biology and Agriculture, National Academy of Sciences, US National Research Council, Publication No. 294, November 1953.
6. *Drinking water and health.* Safe Drinking Water Committee, National Academy of Sciences, US National Research Council, 1977: 372.
7. *Review of fluoride: Benefits and risks.* US Department of Health and Human Services, February 1991: 17.

8. *Health effects of ingested fluoride.* Subcommittee on Health Effects of Ingested Fluoride, Committee on Toxicology, Board on Environmental Studies and Toxicology, Commission on Life Sciences, US National Research Council, August 1993: 128.

9. Kiritsy MC, Levy SM, Warren JJ et al. Assessing fluoride concentrations of juices and juice-flavored drinks. *J Am Dent Assoc* 1996; 127: 895–902.

10. Heilman JR, Kiritsy MC, Levy SM, Wefel JS. Assessing fluoride levels of carbonated soft drinks. *J Am Dent Assoc* 1999; 130: 1593–9.

11. Toumba KJ, Levy S, Curzon ME. The fluoride content of bottled drinking waters. *Br Dent J* 1994; 176: 266–8.

12. Levy SM, Kohout FJ, Guha-Chowdhury N et al. Infants' fluoride intake from drinking water alone, and from water added to formula, beverages, and food. *J Dent Res* 1995: 74: 1399–1407.

13. Yiamouyiannis J. *Fluoride – The aging factor.* 3rd edn. Delaware, OH: Health Action Press, 1993.

14. Stannard JG, Shim YS, Kritsineli M, Labropoulou P, Tsamtsouris A. Fluoride levels and fluoride contamination of fruit juices. *J Clin Pediatr Dent* 1991; 16: 38–40.

15. *Washington Post,* 17 Feb 1999. http://www.washingtonpost.com/wpsrv/national/pesticides.htm.

16. Canadian Conference on the evaluation of current recommendations concerning fluorides, April 9–11, 1992, Fluoride recommendations released. *J Can Dent Assoc* 1993; 59: 330.

17. http://www.ada.org/public/topics/fluoride/artcl-01.html.

18. SM Levy, Kohout FJ, Kiritsy MC, Heilman JR, Wefel JS. Infants' fluoride ingestion from water, supplements and dentifrice. *J Am Dent Assoc* 1995; 126: 1625.

19. Exner FB, Waldbott GL. *The American fluoridation experiment.* New York: Devin-Adair, 1957: 43.

20. Statement by Dr James Patrick before Congressional subcommittee, 4 August 1982. Cited in Null G, Feldman M. *The case against fluoridation*. http://www.garynull.com/documents/fluoride1.htm
21. *Middlesex News*, Natick, MA, Tuesday, 10 March 1998.

5. Fluoride and the Brain

Have you seen the research from China and the USA showing that fluoride is toxic, can damage the central nervous system, and is linked with Alzheimer's disease and low IQ?

BFS suggested answer
Fluoridation is both safe and beneficial. There is no evidence whatsoever to support such claims.

BFS suggested answer refuted
The presence of low levels of fluoride in the drinking water, equal to the amount found in fluoridated water, caused damage to the tissue of the brain similar to Alzheimer's and other forms of dementia, as well as kidney damage.
Dr J.A. Varner et al.[10]

It has been known for many years that fluoride inhibits the enzyme acetylcholinesterase, which is involved in transmitting signals along nerves.[1] Clinical and physiological studies from Russia published in 1974 demonstrated that patients with occupational fluorosis exhibited disturbed nervous activity and brain dysfunction.[2] China, like India, has areas with high levels of endemic fluorosis. Not surprisingly, a great deal of research into other possible adverse effects of fluorides has been conducted in those two countries. The first suggestions that fluoride could affect the brain were published in China in 1982.[3] Since then, many studies have been conducted into the role of fluoride in brain development and its effects on intelligence.

A landmark study

Because it is unethical to subject children to substances known to be toxic, most of the clinical studies with fluorides have been conducted on rats, mice and hamsters. A landmark study was published by Dr Phyllis Mullenix and colleagues in 1995.[4]

Mullenix worked in the Department of Psychiatry at Children's Hospital in Boston and the Department of Neuropathology at Harvard University Medical School. Her studies focussed on neurotoxicity of therapeutic agents: radiation, lead, amphetamine, phenytoin and nitrous oxide, and so on. In 1982 Mullenix was invited by the Director of Forsyth's Dental Infirmary for Children in Boston, Dr John Hein, to conduct research at Forsyth and to apply it to substances used in dentistry. Among those substances, fluoride was prominent.

Until that time, the effects of fluoride on the developing brain had not been considered. Dr Mullenix was to rectify that omission. It was a subject in which she had little interest at the time.

It took until 1986 to complete the computer program they needed for accurate measurement of behaviour in an animal model. The finished program was so perfect that the Forsyth Dental Center was noted for this achievement in the *Wall Street Journal* and the *Boston Herald*.

Mullenix and her team investigated the 'safe and effective' treatment for dental caries by exposing the rats to different concentrations of sodium fluoride (NaF) during late gestation, at weaning and as adults, and by comparing the rats' behaviour and body weight with fluoride levels in their blood and brains. Mullenix expected that rats drinking fluoride-treated water would behave the same as matched, untreated controls – they did not. She had been led to expect that fluoride would not cross the blood/brain barrier, and that if the mothers were fluoridated, the fluoride would not affect the unborn foetus – but in both cases it did. Mullenix says:

'Like walking into quicksand, our confidence that brain function was impervious to fluoride was sinking.'[5]

Published in 1995, the paper by Mullenix and colleagues was the first laboratory study to demonstrate in living animals that the brain was vulnerable to fluoride. They demonstrated that:

- The effects on behaviour depended on the age at exposure.

- Fluoride accumulated in brain tissues.

- The severity of the effect on behaviour increased directly as fluoride levels rose in the blood and the brain.

- Fluoride exposures caused sex- and dose-specific behavioural deficits with a common pattern: males were most sensitive to prenatal exposure, whereas females were more sensitive to weaning and adult exposures.

The fluoride levels used were less than one-tenth the amount found in children one hour after receiving topical applications of dental fluoride gels. Mullenix concluded: 'Thus, humans are being exposed to levels of fluoride we know alters behaviour in rats', levels that 'flagged potential for motor dysfunction, IQ deficits and/or learning disabilities in humans'.

A review by Dr Bruce Spittle of Dunedin School of Medicine, New Zealand, published in 1994,[6] found confirmation in Mullenix's study. Spittle listed case reports that spanned almost sixty years of central nervous system effects in humans excessively exposed to fluoride.

Fluoride and children's IQ

Measuring the intelligence of children aged eight to thirteen years living in areas with no, slight, medium and serious fluorosis, Chinese scientists showed in 1995 that IQ scores were 5–19 points lower for the children in the severe fluorosis area compared with those in the non-fluorosis area.[7] This was confirmed by a second study of children aged seven to fourteen in two areas, one of which had a fluoride level in water four times that of the other (0.91 ppm versus 4.12 ppm).[8] These data, displayed in Figure 1, show a 6–12 point lower IQ in those children from the high-fluoride area compared with those from the low-fluoride area.

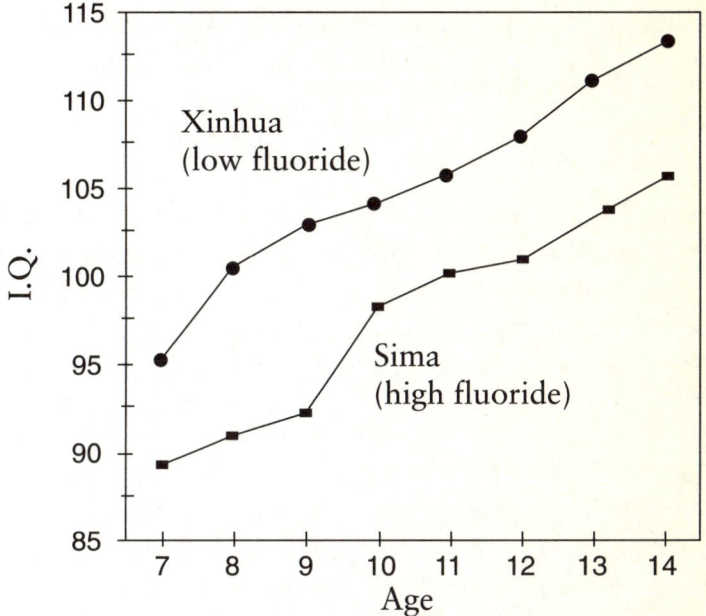

Source: Zhao et al. *Fluoride* 1996; 29: 190–2.

Figure 1. *Comparisons of average IQ by age in Sima and Xinhua*

In this study, intelligence was significantly impaired at a fluoride concentration in drinking water of 4.12 ppm but was not impaired at 0.91 ppm, which is close to the recommended 'optimal' dose. In a study of 8-year-old children, Dr Spittle and colleagues also found no difference in IQ between those drinking water fluoridated at 1 ppm and those whose water contained less than 0.1 ppm. They say: 'Thus a threshold effect for fluoride toxicity may be present with demonstrable effects being present with water containing 4–10 ppm but not 1 ppm of fluoride.'[9]

So should we be worried about water that is fluoridated at 1 ppm? It seems we should if the fluoride comes with other minerals – and in fluoridated tap water, it does. Recent work by Varner and colleagues suggests that fluoride may have the potential to cause neurotoxicity at a level of 1 ppm if present with aluminium ions at a concentration of 0.5 ppm.[10]

Fluoride, aluminium and Alzheimer's disease

For many years, researchers have noticed that elderly people suffering from Alzheimer's disease (senile dementia) have high levels of aluminium in their brains. A large percentage of cookware these days is made of aluminium, and aluminium compounds are frequently added to the water supply as clarifying agents. Are these to blame for the dementia? It's hard, at first sight, to see how, because on its own aluminium is not readily absorbed by the body.

However, add fluoride to the equation, and all that changes: when fluoride is present, it combines with any aluminium to form aluminium fluoride, which is easily absorbed.

After population studies showed a higher incidence of Alzheimer's disease among people who lived in fluoridated areas, Dr Robert Isaacson of the State University of New York added aluminium fluoride to rats' food. He found that the rats lost their sense of smell, developed short-term memory problems and other characteristics of Alzheimer's disease.[11] Dr Mullenix had studied only sodium fluoride. Dr Isaacson's studies compared aluminium fluoride with sodium fluoride to determine if fluoride's effect on aluminium cookware, or its effect when combined with the aluminium sulphate added to some water as a flocculent, had an impact on the development of Alzheimer's disease. It did. The aluminium fluoride was more toxic to the brain than sodium fluoride. This finding has great significance, as Alzheimer's disease was unknown until people started using aluminium cookware.

In January 1987, experiments performed at the Medical Research Endocrinology Department, Newcastle upon Tyne, England, and the Physics Department of the University of Ruhana, Sri Lanka, showed that water 'optimally' fluoridated at 1 ppm, when used in cooking with aluminium cookware, concentrated the aluminium to up to 600 ppm.[12] Fluoridated tap water in Antigo, Wisconsin, in conjunction with aluminium cookware, increased aluminium concentration by 833 times, and the fluoride content doubled.[13]

The maximum aluminium content of water allowed by the World Health Organization is 200 µg per litre. Antigo water, when cooked in aluminium, was seventy-five times over the limit. Dr I. Jansen, who conducted the Antigo study, writes that to 'chance exchanging a hole in a tooth – which can be repaired at a nominal fee – for dementia in later years, for which there is no remedy at any price, hardly seems to be a good bargain'.

Let us also not forget that a large proportion of modern aluminium cookware is lined with a non-stick substance such as Teflon or Tefal, which, made from PTFE (poly-tetra-fluoro-ethane) is another significant source of fluoride.

Fluoride and lead

In 1999 Professor Roger D. Masters of Dartmouth Medical College, and Myron Coplan, a chemical engineer, in a study of 280,000 Massachusetts children found that levels of lead in the blood were significantly higher in communities whose water was fluoridated.[14] Heavy metals compromise normal brain development and neurotransmitter function, leading to long-term deficits in learning and social behaviour. At the individual level, earlier studies revealed that hyperactive children and criminals had significantly elevated levels of lead, manganese or cadmium, compared with controls. High levels of lead in the blood at age seven predicts both juvenile delinquency and adult crime. Surveys of children's blood lead across the United States show that where silicofluorides are used, risk ratios for blood lead over the danger level of 10 µg/dL are up to two and a half times as high as where silicofluorides are not used.

Not surprisingly, communities using silicofluorides report higher rates of learning disabilities, attention deficit disorder (ADD), hyperactivity and violent crime. Data from the US Third National Health and Nutrition Evaluation Survey (NHANES III), and a survey of over 120,000 children in New York towns, corroborate this effect. Masters and Coplan reported that minorities are at particular risk: African-American and Mexican-American children in fluoridated communities have significantly higher levels of lead in their blood than such children in unfluoridated communities.

Ironically, NHANES III also found that children with higher lead levels had more tooth decay.[15] 'So water fluoridation may prove to cause tooth decay rather than prevent it', says lawyer Paul Beeber, president of the New York State Coalition Opposed to Fluoridation.

Lead has long been recognised as having a deleterious effect on the brain. It is for precisely this reason that leaded petrol has been phased out – yet some still insist on adding silicofluorides to drinking water!

Fluoride and hypothyroidism

Fluoride was used for decades as an anti-thyroid medication to treat hyperthyroidism (overactive thyroid). Fluoride is very effective in this context, as it has the ability to mimic the action of TSH – thyroid-stimulating hormone, or thyrotropin. It is highly significant that fluoride was frequently used at levels *below* the current 'optimal' intake of 1 mg/day to suppress the action of the thyroid gland. It should come as no surprise, then, that of the more than 150 symptoms of hypothyroidism (underactive thyroid), almost all are also symptoms of fluoride poisoning.

Canadian thyroid researcher Andreas Schuld, head of a global organisation, Parents of Fluoride-Poisoned Children, found that excessive fluoride intakes correlate with other thyroid-related issues such as iodine deficiency, which is recognised as the most common cause of preventable brain damage and mental disability in the world today.

Fluorine and iodine, both members of the halogen group of elements, have an antagonistic relationship. When there is an excess of fluoride in the body, fluoride competes with iodine and interferes with the function of the thyroid gland. Such interactions affect brain development in the unborn child. Mullenix's observation that those exposed to fluorides before birth were born hyperactive and remained so throughout their lives fits very neatly with existing research on hypothyroidism.

In 1994 another thyroid/fluoride connection was seen in Jennifer Luke's data, which showed that fluoride accumulates in the pineal gland at least as much as, if not more than, in bones and teeth.[16] The pineal gland synthesises melatonin, a hormone that regulates our sleep patterns. Luke showed that melatonin production was inhibited by fluoride in test animals. She also found that this inhibition caused an earlier onset of sexual maturity, an effect already reported in humans in 1956 as part of the Kingston/Newburgh study in New York State. Girls living in fluoridated Newburgh began menstruating significantly earlier than in unfluoridated Kingston.[17]

This early onset of sexual puberty is well established as a symptom of thyroid hormone dysfunction. Usually, patients with low thyroid hormones also have deficient secretion of growth hormone, and may have deficient secretion of the gonadotrophins LH and FSH, which stimulate puberty and reproduction, and ACTH, which is necessary for cortisol and hydrocortisone secretion by the adrenal gland.[18] In this context, it should be noted that aluminium fluoride also mimics the inhibitory action of melatonin.[19]

It is possible that the most common cause of brain damage and mental disability in the world, 'iodine deficiency', could be reduced dramatically simply by reducing fluoride intake.

Fluoride interactions with drugs

Fluoridated pharmaceuticals increase our total fluoride exposure. Antacids, used to treat heartburn and stomach upsets, and probably the world's most prescribed drugs, are aluminium-based. Drugs such as Prozac, designed to act upon the central nervous system, are usually fluoride-based. Both types of drug are so commonly used that they are likely to be taken together, which could have disastrous results in later life. But fluoride in foods and water can also interact with prescribed drugs, with undesirable consequences. With some, fluorides have a synergistic effect, increasing the action of prescribed drugs, while their action on other drugs may have the opposite effect, that of reducing their effectiveness.

Fluoride drugs and violent deaths

Many anti-depressive drugs contain fluoride because of its profound effect on mood. Fluanxol, Motipress, Motival, Parstelin and the biggest seller, Prozac, are all highly fluorinated. Hypothyroidism, which they produce, can induce almost any psychiatric symptom or syndrome, including rage, fear ranging from mild anxiety to frank paranoia, mood swings and aggression.

Recently, the USA has seen an alarming rise in apparently motiveless killings, where individuals – usually men, but also children – have taken a gun and shot several people before shooting themselves.

The number of people, including preschool children, prescribed anti-depressants and stimulants rose in the mid-1990s despite limited knowledge about the effects of such drugs on young children. The reasons for prescribing such medications for young children include pain relief, anxiety associated with medical, pre-surgery and dental procedures, bed-wetting and attention-deficit/hyperactivity disorder in children aged three years and older.

The University of Maryland looked at 200,000 patients in three areas of the country. It found that use of stimulants and anti-depressants rose in all the areas between 1991 and 1995. Julie Zito, principal author of the study, said that some of the drugs' uses are not included in warnings on drug packages. While this is not uncommon with some drugs for adults, there is no information about how these psychotropic drugs work on children: 'Unresolved questions involve the long-term safety of psychotropic medications, particularly in light of earlier ages of initiation and longer durations of treatment.'[20]

In an early case, a young defendant was found not guilty because he committed a murder 'in the course of a hypothyroid psychosis . . . He was later judged to be not guilty by reason of insanity, although he was clearly sane at the time of his trial.'[21]

In a recent rampage, of a kind that has become frighteningly familiar in the USA, Kip Kinkel, a 15-year-old student in Springfield, Oregon, murdered his parents, and the next day ran through a crowded school cafeteria firing his rifle from the hip. He killed two classmates and critically wounded several others. The Associated Press headline read:

> Oregon shooting: Yet another warning of the dangers of Prozac and its clones.[22]

This was disturbingly similar to a violent episode that took place in Louisville, Kentucky, in 1989. Joseph Wesbecker stepped out of an elevator at work, firing an AK-47 semi-automatic assault rifle. Twelve people were wounded and eight killed before Joseph Wesbecker took his own life. One victim described him as 'totally devoid of human element and human soul'.

Kip Kinkel was restrained before he could take his life, but begged others to shoot him when they tackled him. Both he and Wesbecker were taking Prozac at the time of their rampages.

Prozac's manufacturer, Eli Lilly, has repeatedly claimed that Prozac is safe. The International Coalition for Drug Awareness (ICFDA), a non-profit group that warns of potential serious adverse reactions to prescription medications, reports that there is abundant evidence in medical literature showing a link between Prozac and violence, as well as suicide.

Dr Ann Blake Tracy, director of ICFDA, and author of *Prozac: Panacea Or Pandora?*, has testified as an expert witness since 1992 in criminal cases involving Prozac and other anti-depressants. Dr Tracy poses the question: 'How many patients have ever been warned that even something as simple as mixing most major cough syrups with their use of these medications can produce PCP ('angel dust')-like reactions?' 'We are sitting in the middle of this nation's most dangerous drug problem and have not yet awakened to the seriousness of this situation.'[23]

Wesbecker and Kinkel are only two of a growing number of people who commit violent crimes while taking Prozac or one of its clones:

- A mother on Prozac in San Francisco smothered her three small daughters by wrapping their hands and faces with duct tape, and attempted to take her own life.

- A man in Los Angeles on Prozac committed suicide in front of TV cameras.

- A lottery employee taking Luvox (a Prozac clone) in Connecticut shot and killed four fellow workers before taking his own life.

- A man in Wyoming taking Paxil (another Prozac clone) shot and killed his wife, daughter and baby granddaughter before he took his own life.

Many more people have died in similar rampages, and Kinkel is facing a life without his parents and several classmates. He also faces spending the rest of his life in prison while he slowly comes to a realisation of what he did in this drug-induced stupor.

According to internal company documents made public in court cases filed against Eli Lilly, in 1990 they attempted to protect their 'golden goose' (Prozac was bringing in over $6 million per day). Dr Leigh Thompson went 'against the advice of his staff' and told the Board of Directors that suicide and hostile acts committed by Prozac users were, in all probability, caused by the patients' underlying disorders rather than Prozac. On 7 November 1990 he asked, 'What are our priorities?'

Of course priority number one for Eli Lilly was to protect Prozac.

In December 1993 the world heard that Prozac had been found 'not guilty' in the murderous rampage and suicide of Joseph Wesbecker. But in fact, Eli Lilly had paid millions of dollars to settle out of court. The judge was so upset about the secrecy and deception surrounding the case that he called for an additional hearing to force Lilly to admit this publicly. He succeeded, and Lilly and the plaintiffs were forced to admit that this was indeed a settlement and not a 'not guilty' verdict for Prozac.

In another Prozac case against Lilly (*Forsyth* v. *Lilly*) currently being tried in Federal District Court in Hawaii, Judge Alan C. Kay ruled:

- 'Lilly falsified reports of side effects of suicide attempts by reporting them as overdoses.'

- 'Material issues of fact exist as to whether Lilly deliberately suppressed adverse studies.'

- 'The Court finds that Plaintiffs have presented sufficient evidence to show that Lilly may have acted wantonly, oppressively, or with such malice as implies a spirit of mischief or criminal indifference.'

Conclusion

Despite the BFS's denial, there is no doubt that fluoride affects the brain. Why would it be used in drugs that are designed to affect the central nervous system, if it did not? While some effects are considered beneficial, others clearly are not.

These facts alone should be sufficient to limit any individual's exposure to fluoride. *Ad libitum*, unregulated intakes of fluoridated water must pose a risk to the brain.

References

1. Waldbott GL, in collaboration with Burgstahler AW, McKinney HL. *Fluoridation: The great dilemma.* Lawrence, KS: Coronado Press, 1978: 150.

2. Popov LI, Filatova R, Shershever AS. *Gig Tr Prof Zabol* 1974; 5: 25–7. Cited in *Chem Abstr* 1974; 14: 271.

3. Shung-Guan CM et al. The non-skeletal lesions of endemic fluorosis. *Chin J Intern Med* 1982; 21: 217–9. See also: Hu YH. Direct damage on nervous system by fluorosis. Compilation of First Conference on Neuropsychiatric Diseases in Xinjian, China, 1982: 86–8.

4. Mullenix PJ, Denbesten PK, Schunior A, Kernan WJ. Neurotoxicity of sodium fluoride in rats. *J Neurotoxicol Teratol* 1995; 17:169–77.

5. Mullenix PJ. Central nervous system damage from fluorides. 14 September 1998. http://www.cadvision. com/fluoride/brain2.htm. Accessed 13 April 2000.

6. Spittle B. Psychopharmacology of fluoride: a review. *Int Clin Psychopharmacol* 1994; 9: 79–82.

7. Li XS, Zhi JL, Gao RO. Effect of fluoride exposure in intelligence in children. *Fluoride* 1995; 28 (4): 189–92.

8. Zhao LB, Liang G, Zhang D, Lu-Liang XW. Effect of high fluoride water supply on children's intelligence. *Fluoride* 1996; 29 (4): 190–2.

9. Spittle B, Ferguson D, Bouwer C. Intelligence and fluoride exposure in New Zealand children. Abstracts of papers to be presented at the XXIInd Conference of the International Society for Fluoride Research, Bellingham, Washington, USA, 24–27 August 1998: S13.

10. Isaacson RL, Varner JA, Jensen KF. Toxin-induced blood vessel inclusions caused by the chronic administration of aluminium and sodium fluoride and their implications for dementia. Neuroprotective agents. *Ann NY Acad Sci* 1997; 825: 152–66. See also: Varner JA, Jensen KF, Horvath W, Isaacson RL. Chronic administration of aluminium fluoride or sodium fluoride to rats in drinking water: alterations in neuronal and cerebrovascular integrity. *Brain Res* 1998; 784: 284–98.

11. Isaacson, R. Rat studies link brain cell damage with aluminium and fluoride in water. State University of New York, Binghamton, NY. *Wall Street Journal* article by Marilyn Chase, 28 October 1992: B-6.

12. *Sci News* 1987; 131: 73.

13. Jansen I. *J Natl Acad Res Biochem* 1990; Jan/Feb: http:// www.halcyon.com/wfrazier/fluoride.htm.

14. Children's Health and the Environment. 17th International Neurotoxicology Conference, Little Rock, Arkansas, USA, 17–20 October 1999. See also: Masters

RD, Coplan MJ. Water treatment with silicofluorides and lead toxicity. *Int J Environ Studies* 1999; 56: 435–49.

15. Moss ME, Lanphear BP, Auinger P. Association of dental caries and blood lead levels. *J Am Med Assoc* 1999; 281: 2294–8.

16. Luke, JA. Effect of fluoride on the physiology of the pineal gland. *Caries Res* 1994; 28: 204.

17. Schlesinger ER, Overton DE, Chase HC, Cantwell KT. Newburgh–Kingston caries–fluorine study. XIII: Pediatric findings after ten years. *J Am Dent Assoc* 1956; 52: 296–306.

18. Foley, Jr TP. University of Pittsburgh and Children's Hospital of Pittsburgh, Pennsylvania, the MAGIC Foundation Clinical Hypothyroidism Division. http://www.magicfoundation.org/clinhypop.html. Accessed 24 April 2000.

19. Morgan PJ, Hastings MH, Thompson M et al. Intracellular signalling in the ovine pars tuberalis: an investigation using aluminium fluoride and melatonin. *J Mol Endocrinol* 1991; 7: 137–44.

20. Magno Zito, Safer DJ, dosReis S et al. Trends in the prescribing of psychotropic medications to preschoolers. *J Am Med Assoc* 2000; 283: 1025–30.

21. Easson WM. Myxedema psychosis – insanity defense in homicide. *J Clin Psychiatry* 1980; 41: 316–8.

22. http://www.drugawareness.org/oregon.html. Accessed 15 April 2000.

23. Source as in ref. 22.

6. Research into Fluoride

But have *you* read the research?

BFS suggested answer
One needs to be an expert in very specialised fields of medicine to be able to assess the validity of such papers. I know that scientists who are recognised experts in the relevant disciplines have reviewed these papers and found that they are not relevant to water fluoridation.

BFS suggested answer refuted
Most of what you think you know about fluoride just isn't so. Consider the facts, check the references, and dare to think.
Darlene Sherrell, 1997

As I mentioned previously, my dentist, a university lecturer on dentistry, admitted knowing nothing about fluoride and relying entirely on other 'experts'.

Throughout the history of fluoridation, there has been widespread reliance on the words of others and a failure to investigate reports of adverse effects of fluoride. This lack of willingness to investigate is not just a failure of individual scientists, doctors and dentists: it extends to the US public health service, which was involved in the early trials, accepted the findings of those trials unreservedly, and subsequently poured millions of dollars into promoting fluoridation; and to British and Irish government 'health authorities', whose brief is supposedly to protect the public health.

The second sentence of the BFS's suggested answer is true – in a way. Much of the research done in the early days isn't relevant to water fluoridation today – it was conducted using calcium fluoride or sodium fluoride, which bear little resemblance to the silicofluorides that are put in drinking water.

The first sentence of the BFS answer is just as worrying. I have no paper qualifications in either dentistry or chemistry, but I have no difficulty whatsoever understanding the findings of the hundreds of papers I have read. If I come across a word I don't understand, I consult my medical dictionary. Surely dentists, whom we expect to know about such things, should understand them?

The last worry, which is an even bigger one, is that unelected health authorities currently make the decision on whether to fluoridate their respective areas, and if the New Labour government in the UK has its way, that responsibility will be devolved to local councils. This means that two bodies that are unlikely to have any first-hand knowledge whatsoever about the relative merits or dangers of fluoridation have the sole responsibility for mass medicating whole populations without their consent – something no doctor can legally do.

And it's all based on what somebody else says, because nobody on the pro-fluoridation side seems willing to read the research, and, judging by the BFS answer, pro-fluoridationists do not feel that they are capable of understanding that research if they did read it.

A dentist finds out for himself

All dentists aren't so medically illiterate. Here is a true story of one dentist who could understand the research, pursued it, and came out against fluoridation as a result.

Don MacAuley was a young dentist practising in Dublin, Ireland. Like most in his profession, he believed what he had been taught at college: that fluoride was a safe and effective defence against dental decay. His patients, however, voiced concerns. They asked him why, when the rest of Europe was so strongly opposed to fluoridation, Ireland was alone in endorsing it. Wanting to allay his patients' concerns, he promised to make some investigations. When he studied the volume of international medical literature on fluoridation, he discovered that the fluoride story had a sinister side, of which he was unaware:

- Irish dentists told him that up to 40 per cent of Irish people suffered from dental fluorosis; that up to 80 per cent of children in fluoridated North America also had the condition.

- This mottling or staining of the teeth meant that too much of the chemical was present in the body; Canadian dental authorities conceded that fluoride could lead to bone and tooth destruction and could damage overall health; foreign research linked fluoride to hip fracture, bone disease, brain disorders and irritable bowel syndrome.

- Dr Hardy Limeback, professor of preventive dentistry at Toronto University and consultant to the Canadian Dental Authority, claimed that water fluoridation had actually contributed to the birth of the multimillion-pound cosmetic dentistry industry; that more money was being spent treating dental fluorosis than would be spent on dental caries if water were not fluoridated.

MacAuley found confirmation of these claims in his own knowledge, so he sought guidance, correctly, from the Irish Dental Association, his governing body.

'To my surprise, I never received a reply', he says.

I wrote two letters outlining the worries of my patients and stating I had a moral obligation to give them answers, but I heard nothing. I also wrote to the Chief Dental Officer at the Department of Health and was sent a fact sheet on Irish dental policy and the website address of the American Dental Association. This provided no information on the situation in Ireland.

Using the Freedom of Information Act, MacAuley requested details of research that had been done in Ireland on the effects of fluoride on public health, a stipulation under the Health (Fluoridation of Water Supplies) Act 1960. He also asked about the type and amount of fluoride used in Irish water, and where it came from.

The Irish Department of Health referred him to the regional health boards. He wrote to all eight. The next week, MacAuley received a telephone call from a senior dental surgeon at a health board outside his locality. The surgeon asked the reason for his questions, whether he planned to publish the results – and what his political affiliations were! He received telephone calls from other health board officials urging him to withdraw his Freedom of Information request and conform to Irish Dental Association policy. He says: 'I was completely amazed. I couldn't believe that the details of what I thought was a confidential request had been revealed. I contacted my solicitor who advised me to persevere with my enquiries.'

Four weeks later, he received guarded replies from several health boards. The Southern Health Board told him to look for answers he wanted in the library. 'I felt there was an increasing resistance from officialdom to respond to my questions, but I was determined to get to the bottom of it.'

Eventually, MacAuley appealed to the Information Commissioner. After waiting almost a year, he finally received answers that confirmed his fears. He learned:

- that the fluoridating agent used in drinking water in Ireland, hydrofluorosilicic acid, was a non-biodegradable, highly corrosive substance, contaminated with a number of toxic substances, including arsenic;

- that according to reports by the Environmental Protection Agency in 1997, 9 per cent of all water supplies in Ireland exceeded the recommended levels of 1 mg fluoride per litre of water – which is illegal and impermissible;

- that in thirty-five years of fluoridation, no Irish government had ever carried out a public health survey on its effects.

By now, MacAuley was convinced that the Irish public was being denied the truth; that there was a hidden agenda to reveal as little as possible about fluoridation.

At dental school, you are taught only one side of the story, and if dentists don't know the full story, how can our patients be expected to. Water fluoridation is sold as the greatest preventive oral health measure ever devised, but the story is biased and the indoctrination manipulative. In my view, many dentists continue to endorse fluoridation simply because they do not know the truth. They are not told that the fluoride used here is toxic waste contaminated with arsenic and lead. They are not told there is enough fluoride in a tube of toothpaste to kill a small child or that, according to the US Environmental Protection Agency, it is more poisonous than lead. Yet we are expected to accept that a toxic waste diluted in our drinking water is safe.

The whole episode has been both shocking and emotionally draining. It is amazing the lengths to which proponents of fluoridation will go to protect this pollutant. If the government continues to mass medicate the Irish public without its consent, it will inevitably have to face up to the consequences. When it does, it is my belief that the bill to the taxpayer will dwarf the army deafness claims.

Don MacAuley is now firmly against fluoride. He now has a private practice and acts as advisor to the Irish Fluoride Free

Water campaign. He is determined to educate his patients and colleagues about the truth behind fluoridation.

The Irish government breaks its own law

In a recent interview, the Irish Minister for Health, Micheál Martin, said that the reason the Irish government had never carried out a public health survey on the effects of fluoridation that its own law, the Health (Fluoridation of Water Supplies) Act 1960, requires, was that the population of Ireland was 'too small'.[1]

Dentists obviously are not experts

In Britain, frustrated by the apparent lack of progress in getting more water fluoridated, the British Fluoridation Society and NHS started promoting the supply of fluoridated milk early in 2001.[2]

This action is a prime illustration of the BFS's lack of understanding of the science of fluoridation:

- Because fluoride is a cumulative poison, the WHO website states very clearly that analysis of children's urine should be considered mandatory for safety reasons when programmes to fluoridate school milk are introduced. They say, 'Dental and public health administrators should be aware of the total fluoride exposure in the population before introducing any additional fluoride programme for caries prevention.'[3] The BFS seems unaware of such warnings or, indeed, of the need for them.

- But — and this is the telling part — they do not realise that when sodium fluoride is added to milk it reacts with the calcium and precipitates out calcium fluoride, which sinks to the bottom of the glass within one hour.

They do not know that if the milk has been stored for any length of time children will absorb very little, if any, of it. They also appear not to appreciate that calcium fluoride is not easily absorbed from the gut. Or that, according to the US Academy of Sciences, 'Calcium rich foods cause elimination of systemic fluoride in faeces equal to or greater than the fluoride intake'.[4] It is for these reasons that instructions on fluoride supplements state that the supplements should not be taken with milk. They also explain why toxicologists recommend milk in order to minimise the effects of fluoride poisoning. So, if you want children to absorb fluoride, the last thing you should put it in is milk.

Conclusion

If dentists declare they know of nothing adverse about the effects of fluoride, this is a reflection not of the state of science on the matter, but of their own arrogant indolence.

References

1. Fluoride in our water: are we brushing with danger? *Irish Independent*, 29 March 2000.
2. Children to get fluoride in school milk, *The Independent*, 21 January 2001.
3. WHO Geneva: World Health Organization, *Fluorides and dental health*, 1994.
4. Standing Committee on the Scientific Evaluation of Dietary Reference Intakes, Food and Nutrition Board, Institute of Medicine *Dietary reference intakes for calcium, phosphorus, magnesium, vitamin D and fluoride*, Washington, DC: National Academy Press, 1999.

7. Fluoridation and High Infant Mortality

> Do you know that in Chile fluoridation was stopped after ten years because of Dr Schatz's work, which linked fluoridation to high infant mortality – particularly among under-nourished children?

BFS suggested answer

At present around 5 million people in Chile drink fluoridated water, and we understand that the Chile Government intends to extend coverage to the whole population. Fluoridation in Chile was suspended in the 1970s at a time of great political unrest. It was reinstated in 1985.

BFS suggested answer refuted

Fluoridation is the greatest fraud that has ever been perpetrated, and it has been perpetrated on more people than any other fraud has.
Professor Albert Schatz, 1982

Dr Albert Schatz is probably best known for his discovery of the antibiotic streptomycin, the first antibiotic to be effective in the treatment of tuberculosis.

Between 1962 and 1965, Schatz and his family lived in Chile, where he was a professor in the Faculties of Medicine, of Chemistry and Pharmacy, of Agronomy, of Odontology and of Philosophy and Education at the University of Chile. He was also a member of the Rector's Advisory Staff at the University of Chile and helped reorganise research and scientific teaching in that country. In addition, he was associated with projects at the Chilean Ministries of Health, Agronomy and Education; at the University of Conception and Catholic University; and with UNESCO and the Food and Agriculture Organization. In November 1965, the University of Chile awarded him an honorary degree for his contributions to that country.

Dr Schatz investigated the relationship between artificial fluoridation and increased death rates in Chile. He says he chose Chile for his research because pro-fluoridationists had never adequately studied the effect of fluoridation on poor, malnourished people as a specific group.

Using officially collected data, it soon became obvious to Schatz that fluoride was having a devastating effect. For example, Curico, which was fluoridated, had almost two and a half times as many deaths of children with congenital malformations as non-fluoridated San Fernando, and nearly three times more such deaths than the country of Chile taken as a whole.[1] His research on fluoridation in Chile demonstrated that malnourished infants are the most susceptible to fluoride toxicity (see also Chapter 20).

In 1964 Schatz wrote to Dr Leland C. Hendershot, the editor of the *Journal of the American Dental Association*, with a view to publishing his findings. He received no reply. In the first three months of 1965, Schatz wrote three more letters to *JADA*, in which he discussed his evidence of the frightening consequences of fluoridation. *All three letters were refused and returned to him unopened.* In other words, Hendershot, on behalf of the American Dental Association, had rejected the findings of a world-renowned Nobel Prize-winning scientist out of hand without even the courtesy of opening the letters and reading them. It is one of the most blatant cases of censorship in scientific history.

Schatz says: 'Such a response is typical of the proponents of fluoridation. The professional sanctions for opposing fluoridation can be severe, and it is best not to even acknowledge evidence of harm or ineffectiveness.'

In 1993 Schatz attested to the high levels of infant mortality in Chile after drinking water was fluoridated in that country. The following are some of the statements he made in his affidavit:[2]

> In Chile, with widespread malnutrition and high infant mortality, it was not necessary to observe a generation of people throughout their entire lifespan in order to determine whether artificial fluoridation is or is not harmful. One could see the lethal effect of fluoridation within the first year of life in terms of increased infant mortality due to acute toxicity of fluoride.
>
> In the US, the harmful effects of artificial fluoridation are not so clearly revealed . . . because Americans as a whole are in a considerably better state of nutrition than Chileans.
>
> Nonetheless, artificial fluoridation of drinking water may well dwarf the thalidomide tragedy . . . Many victims of artificial fluoridation . . . die quietly during the first year of their lives, or at a later age under conditions where their deaths are attributed to some other cause.

Salvador Allende was President of Chile from his election on 4 September 1970 until his assassination by a military junta on 11 September 1973. Allende was more than a president; as a medical doctor, he was concerned about the poor people of Chile. It is well known that calcium protects against fluoride. The consumption of milk, which is the major source of calcium for infants, is especially important. On his election, Allende initiated a government programme under which free milk was delivered daily to pregnant and nursing mothers, and to children under the age of fifteen.[3] At that time, Schatz says, 'half the children in Chile under 15 years were undernourished, and 600,000 were mentally retarded through lack of protein, especially during the first months of life'. This was the health of half the children fluoridated in Chile in the 1960s. During Allende's short presidency, birth weight of babies increased for the first time in fifty years, and, as a result of Schatz's work, fluoridation was stopped in Chile.

Today, according to WHO figures, about 10 per cent of a Chilean population of 14.3 million again drink fluoridated water. That's fewer than 1.5 million people – not 5 million, as claimed by the British Fluoridation Society.

Table 1 shows decayed, missing and filled teeth (DMFT) and fluoride in drinking water in various Chilean cities.[4] In terms of DMFT the figures may look good, but overall the difference between the most and least fluoridated cities is less than 2.5 teeth – and look at the rates of fluorosis.

City	Fluoride conc. (ppm)	DMFT	% Fluorosis
Rancagua	0.07	5.06	6.7
Santiago	0.21	4.12	7.4
La Serena	0.55	3.55	16.5
San Felipe	0.93	3.33	25.3
Iquique	1.10 (natural)	2.60	56.8

Source: WHO Oral Health Country/Area Profile Programme, Department of Noncommunicable Diseases Surveillance/Oral Health, WHO Collaborating Centre, Malmö University, Sweden.

Table 1. DMFT and fluorosis among 15-year-olds at various sites in Chile

Conclusion

Since fluoride was reintroduced into Chile in 1985, according to the WHO statistics, the trend in dental decay has increased. The average DMFT in 12-year-olds in 1989 was 6.0. In 1991 it had fallen to 5.3, but by 1995 the numbers were up to 6.7. This suggests that DMFT had been falling before fluoridation was reintroduced, but that the fall was reversed by the fluoride. These figures and the high incidence of fluorosis in Chile demonstrate that fluoridation is not improving dental health in that country – rather the reverse.

References

1. Schatz A. *Low-level fluoridation and low-level radiation: Two case histories of misconduct in science.* Schatz, Philadelphia, PA, 1996.
2. Schatz A. Affidavit in support of motion for summary judgement, Circuit Court, Fond du Lac County, Wisconsin.
3. Schatz, A. Increased death rates in Chile associated with artificial fluoridation of drinking water, with implications for other countries. *J Arts Sci Humanities* 1976; 2: 1–17.
4. WHO Oral Health Country/Area Profile Programme, Department of Noncommunicable Diseases Surveillance/ Oral Health, WHO Collaborating Centre, Malmö University, Sweden, 1995.

8. Fluoride as a Cumulative Poison

Do you agree that fluoride is a cumulative poison that is more toxic than lead/arsenic?

BFS suggested answer

We do not agree. Water fluoridation is both safe and beneficial. It involves adjusting the naturally occurring level of fluoride to that which we know benefits dental health – 1 part of fluoride per million parts of water.

BFS suggested answer refuted

Fluoride is an accumulative poison which accumulates in the skeletal structures, including the teeth, when the body is exposed to small daily intakes of this element . . . it is like lead accumulation in the bone until saturation occurs and then lead poisoning sets in.
Dr P.H. Phillips, biochemist, University of Wisconsin

Dentists know that fluoride is toxic . . .

One has to wonder at the brazen cheek of the BFS's suggested answer. How can dentists deny both that fluorides are as toxic as lead and arsenic and that the effect is cumulative, or claim that they are unaware of those facts, when it was the *Journal of the American Dental Association*, no less, that first made this statement in 1936? It said: 'Fluoride at the 1 ppm concentration is as toxic as arsenic and lead . . . there is an increasing volume of evidence of the injurious effects of fluorine, especially the chronic intoxication resulting from the ingestion of minute amounts of fluorine over long period of time."[1]

Other extracts from this paper illustrate clearly that before the first city was fluoridated, the dental profession took a very dim view of fluoride. In fact, dentists were all in favour of removing as much fluoride from water as they could:

> The studies conducted by Dr Smith and her co-workers at the University of Arizona have shown that 1 ppm, and possibly 0.8 ppm, of fluorine will produce definite signs of enamel dystrophy in children born and reared in an endemic area.
>
> . . . a comparison of toxicity data suggests that fluorine, lead and arsenic belong to the same group, as far as ability to cause some symptom of toxicity in minute dosage is concerned.
>
> Fluorine, a general protoplasmic poison, exerts a strong inhibitory action on many enzymes. The more complex inorganic compounds containing fluorine are frequently toxic because of a direct action of the compound itself, or because of a conversion of the complex compound, as by hydrolysis [changing by taking up the elements of water], into simpler compounds, such as the simpler fluorides.

Despite such valid early studies, American Dental Association and US public health service literature today emphatically indicates that as long as your teeth are free of cavities, the longevity of the rest of your body is irrelevant.

. . . and so do doctors . . .

In 1942, before the first city was fluoridated, the editor of the prestigious *Journal of the American Medical Association* told his readers:

> Fluorides are general protoplasmic poisons, probably because of their capacity to modify the metabolism of

cells by changing the permeability of the cell membrane and by inhibiting certain enzyme systems . . . The sources of fluorine intoxication are drinking water containing 1 part per million or more of fluorine, fluoride compounds used as insecticidal sprays for fruits and vegetables (cryolite and barium fluosilicate) and the mining and conversion of phosphate rock to superphosphate, which is used as fertilizer.[2]

So doctors knew too. They also knew about the fertiliser connection, which, ironically, was to play such a big part in water fluoridation in years to come.

. . . even pharmacists know

More recently, the *US Dispensary*,[3] a reference book used by pharmacists, states:

[F]luorides are violent poisons to all living tissue because of their precipitation of calcium. They cause a fall in blood pressure, respiratory failure and general paralysis. Continuous ingestion of nonfatal doses (as in the water supply and fluoride in toothpaste) causes permanent inhibition of growth.

In yet another reference text book, the *Clinical Toxicology of Commercial Products: Acute Poisoning*, lead is given a toxicity rating of 3 to 4, while fluoride is rated at 4 (3 = moderately toxic, 4 = very toxic). The authors say: 'The fact is that fluoride is more toxic than lead and just slightly less toxic than arsenic.'[4]

A committee of the National Research Council of Canada declared:

Fluoride is a persistent bioaccumulator, and is entering into human food and beverage chains in increasing amounts. Careful consideration of all available data indicates that the amount of fluoride ingested daily in foods and beverages by adult humans living in fluoridated communities currently ranges between 3.5 and 5.5 mg . . . Long-term ingestion, with accumulation of fluoride in animals and man, induces metabolic and biochemical changes . . . It cannot be assumed that such changes are of no significance to human health . . . fluoride has displayed mutagenic activity in studies of vegetation, insects, and mammalian oocytes. There is a high correlation between carcinogenicity and mutagenicity of pollutants, and fluoride has been one of the major pollutants in several situations where a high incidence of respiratory cancer has been observed.[5]

Conclusion

This evidence of prior knowledge by the dental profession gives the lie to the BFS's answer. The evidence dentists themselves cite should be enough to satisfy any sane person that fluorides are extremely toxic and that their adverse effects increase with time. Nevertheless, on 7 December 1992, the US Environmental Protection Agency set the maximum contaminant level (MCL) for lead at 0.015 ppm, with a goal of getting rid of it altogether. Yet the MCL for fluoride is currently set at 4.0 ppm – some 266 times as high. How does this make sense?

References

1. Editorial. Fluoride is not an essential nutrient. *J Am Dent Assoc* 1936; 23: 568–74.
2. Editorial. Chronic fluorine intoxication. *J Am Med Assoc* 1943; 123: 150.
3. *US Dispensary*. 24th ed, 1950, pp 1456–7.

4. Ambiance J. *The clinical toxicology of commercial products: Acute poisoning.* 5th edn. Baltimore, MD: Williams and Wilkins, 1984.
5. Associate Committee On Scientific Criteria for Environmental Quality. *Environmental fluoride.* NRCC No. 16081. National Research Council of Canada, 1977.

9. Fluoride Kills

Is it true that there is enough fluoride in a tube of toothpaste to kill a small child?

BFS suggested answer

Used sensibly, fluoride toothpaste presents no risks to children. Fluoride toothpaste has brought about massive improvements in dental health since its introduction in the early 1970s. Everyone – children and adults – should brush their teeth thoroughly with an appropriate fluoride toothpaste twice a day. Parents of children under the age of 7 should supervise children's brushing and use a small pea-sized amount or a smear of toothpaste. Children should be encouraged to spit out excess toothpaste.

BFS suggested answer refuted

The Nassau County toxicologist testified that the amount of fluoride put on William's teeth, which he subsequently swallowed was three times the amount needed to be fatal. The court awarded damages of $750,000.
New York Times, 20 January 1979

There are many conditions attributed to fluoride intake that increase death rates by damaging the immune system or promoting conditions such as osteoporosis. That fluoride is responsible is hotly debated. But there have been some cases of death where there is no dispute. Fluoride can kill.

Why don't dentists need to know . . .

According to dentists, fluorides are safe – but what do they know? The following advice was given to British dentists on page 300 of the 15 September 1970 issue of the *British Dental Journal*. It advised its readers:

> Perhaps the greatest deterrent to meaningful political engagement of dentists in the promotion of water fluoridation is the mistaken but widespread assumption that to do so they must have full and complete knowledge of the detailed and voluminous scientific literature on the relationship of water fluoridation to dental and general health. They do not . . . as soon as dentists recognise their responsibility in the politics of fluoridation, their performance will be outstanding. In politics, the emphasis is on propagandising rather than education.

Consider also this statement by the American Dental Association in 1979:

> Individual dentists must be convinced that they need not be familiar with scientific reports and field investigations on fluoridation to be effective participants and that non-participation is overt neglect of personal responsibility.

. . . that fluoride can kill

If dentists do not have to know about possible side effects of fluoride, how can they possibly expect to give informed guidance to their patients on its use? It is precisely because a dentist was unaware that fluoride was toxic that a young boy died in 1974 after having his teeth cleaned. The resultant court case was reported in the 20 January 1979 edition of the *New York Times*.

The 3-year-old boy, William Kennerly, was taken to the dentist for a routine checkup. No caries was found and the boy was handed over to the hygienist for a routine tooth cleaning. After this, the boy's teeth were swabbed with a fluoride gel. He was then given a glass of water to swill out his mouth. As he was not instructed to spit it out, he swallowed it.

> William began vomiting, sweating and complaining of headache and dizziness. His mother, appealing to the dentist, was told that the child had only been given routine treatment. But she was not satisfied, and was sent to the Brookdale Ambulatory Pediatric Care unit in the same building.

After waiting for two and a half hours, while his mother continually appealed for help, the child lapsed into a coma, had adrenalin pumped into his heart to revive him and was taken to a nearby hospital. Here, after another wait of over an hour, William lapsed back into a coma and died.

The Nassau County toxicologist testified that the amount of fluoride put on William's teeth, which he subsequently swallowed, was *three times the amount needed to be fatal*. The court awarded damages of $750,000.

This case is not an isolated one either in the USA or the rest of the world.

Although the BFS seems unconcerned about possible risks to infants of ingesting toothpaste, the danger to children is taken seriously by some. On 2 March 1999, a new packaging rule came into force in the USA. The Consumer Product Safety Commission issued a rule requiring all household products containing more than 50 mg or 0.5 per cent elemental fluoride to be packed in child-proof containers 'to protect children under 5 years of age from serious personal injury and serious illness resulting from handling or ingesting a toxic amount of elemental fluoride'.[1]

It is significant that, under this rule, commodities such as 'safe' fluoridated toothpaste and tea will also have to be so packaged.

In Canada, Parents of Fluoride-Poisoned Children commissioned a government-approved laboratory to test for the fluoride content of tea.[2] The test showed a soluble elemental fluorine content of 69 ppm in black tea (1 teabag + 8 ounces of fluid) and 88 ppm in green tea. That is 17.25 mg and 22 mg per cup, respectively. Based on these data, it should be clear that, even under normal living conditions, merely drinking one cup of tea is highly risky.

References

1. Consumer Product Safety Commission, 16 CFR, Part 1700, Final rule: Requirements for child-resistant packaging; Household products with more than 50 mg of elemental fluoride and more than 0.5 per cent elemental fluoride; and Modification of exemption for oral prescription drugs with sodium fluoride. 63 *Fed Reg* 105 (2 June 1998).

2. Schuld A (Parents of Fluoride-Poisoned Children). Reply to Dr Coggon, http://www.bruha.com/fluoride/html/reply_to_dr._coggon.htm. Accessed 11 February 2000.

10. People at Risk from Fluoride

Is fluoridated water safe for people with certain medical conditions, such as diabetes or kidney failure?

BFS suggested answer
Yes. Fluoridated water is safe for everyone to drink. There is no evidence that drinking fluoridated water is harmful to anyone irrespective of their state of health.

BFS suggested answer refuted
Subsets of the population may be unusually susceptible to the toxic effects of fluoride and its compounds. These populations include the elderly, people with deficiencies of calcium, magnesium, and/or vitamin C, and people with cardiovascular and kidney problems.
US Agency for Toxic Substances and Disease Registry, 1993

It was known over a quarter of a century ago that some people are more susceptible to the adverse effects of fluoride than others. In 1972, the *Journal of the American Medical Association* published a paper on the effects of fluoride in people with impaired kidney function. It read:

> Children, the elderly and any person with impaired kidney function [which includes many AIDS patients], are in the high risk group for fluoride poisoning and must be warned to monitor their fluoride intake. Also at high risk are people with immunodeficiencies, diabetes and heart ailments, as well as anyone with calcium, magnesium and Vitamin C deficiencies. At the level of

0.4 ppm renal [kidney] impairment has been shown.[1] [Note that 0.4 ppm is less than half the 'optimal' amount that is put in drinking water.]

Five years later, another researcher published similar findings, saying:

. . . the ever-increasing use (and release) of fluoride compounds in the environment should be of long-term concern in population sub-groups who are most susceptible, and therefore, most at risk. One of these sub-groups consists of people with impaired kidney function, including subjects with nephropathic diabetes. The diabetes factor is of particular relevance, not only because the incidence of diabetes has increased by 6%/yr during the period 1965–1975, but also because subjects with nephropathic diabetes can exhibit a polydipsia–polyurea syndrome that results in increased intake of fluoride, along with greater-than-normal retention of a given fluoride dosage. People with inadequate dietary intakes (particularly of [Calcium] and/or Vitamin C) are also likely to be more at risk as a consequence of low-dose long-term fluoride ingestion.[2]

In the same year, the US National Academy of Sciences warned:

. . . renal patients have a lower margin of safety than the average person . . . One case of symptomatic skeletal fluorosis (radiculomyelopathy) has been reported from an area in Texas with natural fluoride at 2.3–3.5 ppm in the water (1965). There have been two cases of suspected skeletal fluorosis . . . The combination of renal impairment and very high water intake were thought to account for these findings.[3]

That made it official.

Over the years reports kept coming in about fluoridated water causing health problems for those whose health was poor. It particularly affected anyone whose system was unable to rid the body of ingested fluoride or whose general nutrient intake was poor. In most of these cases, it was the poorer and more disadvantaged elements in society who were worst affected.

In 1993, the US Agency for Toxic Substances and Disease Registry reiterated:

> Existing data indicate that subsets of the population may be unusually susceptible to the toxic effects of fluoride and its compounds. These populations include the elderly, people with deficiencies of calcium, magnesium, and/or vitamin C, and people with cardiovascular and kidney problems . . . Because fluoride is excreted through the kidney, people with renal insufficiency would have impaired renal clearance of fluoride. Impaired renal clearance of fluoride has also been found in people with diabetes mellitus and cardiac insufficiency. People over the age of 50 often have decreased renal fluoride clearance . . . This decreased clearance of fluoride may indicate that elderly people are more susceptible to fluoride toxicity . . . Because of the role of calcium in bone formation, calcium deficiency would be expected to increase susceptibility to effects of fluoride.[4]

Drink mineral water instead?

Many people drink mineral water, at vastly inflated prices, precisely in an effort to avoid impurities believed to be present in tap water. In 1986, a French medical journal reported skeletal fluorosis in patients with impaired kidney function who drank the French mineral water Vichy Saint-Yorre, which has a particularly high calcium fluoride content. The paper concludes: '[T]he prolonged administration of Vichy Saint-

Yorre water containing 8.5 mg of fluoride ion per liter, provokes a skeletal fluorosis. This intoxication appeared very quickly if the patient suffered from an even mild renal failure.'[5]

The difficulty now is that, as the fluoride content is generally not stated on bottles of mineral water and may be inaccurate even when it is, those attempting to avoid fluoridated tap water may not be able to do so.

Dialysis is dodgy

On 30 August 2000, one dialysis patient died and sixteen were hospitalised after being treated at dialysis centres in Youngstown, Ohio, in the United States. It was the latest in a long list of such disasters. Sam Brooks, chairman and chief executive officer of Renal Care Group, which runs the centres, said: 'They got very ill, were nauseous and throwing up and our medical director immediately shut down the water system because when something like this happens, it's most likely [the fault of] the water system.'[6] The cause of this accident is under investigation, but there have been similar instances in which malfunctions in the dialysis machines, resulting in the patients' taking in fluoridated water, were found to be the cause. Here are just two.

On 16 July 1993, fluoride poisoning was blamed for the deaths of three dialysis patients at the University of Chicago Hospitals. Spokeswoman Susan Phillips said symptoms suffered by the victims, and by six other dialysis patients who developed symptoms similar to allergic reactions, 'were consistent with fluoride exposure'. Traces of the chemical were found in patients' blood and in water samples. As the *Chicago Sun-Times* noted, water standards in the USA are based on exposure in healthy people to 14 litres per week – but dialysis patients use more than 300 litres per week.[7]

A dialysis patient died in Annapolis, Maryland, in November 1979. Other dialysis patients suffered cardiac arrest, nausea, hypotension, chest pain, diarrhoea, itching, flushing, vomiting, difficult breathing, profuse sweating, weakness, numbness, and stomach cramping. Water consumers not on dialysis also reported nausea, headache, cramps, diarrhoea and dizziness.[8] This was caused by a malfunction of the fluoridation equipment that released fluoride into the drinking water. 'Even though state and county health officials learned of the spill . . . no public announcement was made and the City Council was not told of the situation for six more days.' A county health officer said that the delay in notification was because '[w]e didn't want to jeopardise the fluoridation program'.[9]

Conclusion

Despite the BFS's cavalier answer, which is either a display of crass ignorance or of wilful deceit, it is no secret that fluoridated water is *not* 'safe for everyone to drink'. There is no justification to take chances with a whole population, which includes people who are known to be particularly vulnerable or sensitive to fluoride. No risk is acceptable if it is avoidable.

The BFS is funded by government. Is it not the responsibility of government and health authorities to protect the vulnerable in our society from such unnecessary risks?

References

1. Juncos LI, Donadio JV. Renal failure and fluorosis, fluorine and dental health. *J Am Med Assoc* 1972; 222 (7): 783–5.
2. Marier JR. Some current aspects of environmental fluoride. *Sci Total Environ* 1977; November: 253–65.
3. *Drinking water and health*. Safe Drinking Water Committee, National Academy of Sciences, US National Research Council, 1977: 380.

4. *Toxicological profile for fluorides, hydrogen fluoride, and fluorine (F)*. US Department of Health and Human Services, Agency for Toxic Substances and Disease Registry, April 1993: 112.

5. Boivin G, Chavassieux P, Chapuy MC, Baud CA, Meunier PJ. Histomorphometric profile of bone fluorosis induced by prolonged ingestion of Vichy Saint-Yorre water. Comparison with bone fluorine levels. *Pathol Biol* (Paris), 1986; 34: 33–9.

6. Man dies after dialysis treatment: 16 people hospitalized from problems caused at Youngstown center. *Akron Beacon Journal*, 2 September 2000.

7. Fluoride blamed in 3 deaths: Traces found in blood of U. of C. dialysis patients. *Chicago Sun-Times*, 31 July 1993.

8. Fluoride linked to death. *Evening Capital*, Annapolis, MD, 29 November 1979.

9. Middletown, Maryland, latest city to receive toxic spill of fluoride in their drinking water. *Townsend Letter for Doctors* 1994; 135: 1124–6.

11. EPA Scientists and Fluoride

Is it true that scientists at the American Environmental Protection Agency have found that fluoridated water causes an alarming number of health problems and should be stopped?

BFS suggested answer

No. The EPA supports the US Public Health Service policy of fluoridation. The EPA is the official Government body in the USA which sets the maximum level for fluoride in water. (Similar to the Department of the Environment in the UK).

BFS suggested answer refuted

EPA professionals were never asked to conduct a thorough, independent analysis of the fluoride literature. Instead, their credentials were used to give the appearance of scientific credibility. They were used to support the predetermined conclusion that 4 mg/l of fluoride in drinking water was safe.
Dr Robert Carton, former EPA environmental scientist

The BFS's suggested answer doesn't answer the question that was asked. The truthful answer to that is: Yes, it is true. In May 1999, the EPA's 1,500 scientists voted to oppose the fluoridation of drinking water supplies. This is their statement, published with permission.

Statement prepared on behalf of the National Treasury Employees Union Chapter 280 by Chapter senior vice-president J. William Hirzy, PhD, May 1, 1999

The following documents why our union, formerly

National Federation of Federal Employees Local 2050 and since April 1998 Chapter 280 of the National Treasury Employees Union, took the stand it did opposing fluoridation of drinking water supplies. Our union is comprised of [sic] and represents the approximately 1500 scientists, lawyers, engineers and other professional employees at EPA Headquarters here in Washington, DC. The union first became interested in this issue rather by accident. Like most Americans, including many physicians and dentists, most of our members had thought that fluoride's only effects were beneficial – reductions in tooth decay, etc. We too believed assurances of safety and effectiveness of water fluoridation.

Then, as EPA was engaged in revising its drinking water standard for fluoride in 1985, an employee came to the union with a complaint: he said he was being forced to write into the regulation a statement to the effect that EPA thought it was alright for children to have 'funky' teeth. It was OK, EPA said, because it considered that condition to be only a cosmetic effect, not an adverse health effect. The reason for this EPA position was that it was under political pressure to set its health-based standard for fluoride at 4 mg/liter. At that level, EPA knew that a significant number of children develop moderate to severe dental fluorosis, but since it had deemed the effect as only cosmetic, EPA didn't have to set its health-based standard at a lower level to prevent it.

We tried to settle this ethics issue quietly, within the family, but EPA was unable or unwilling to resist external political pressure, and we took the fight public with a union amicus curiae brief in a lawsuit filed against EPA by a public interest group. The union has published on this initial involvement period in detail.[1]

Since then our opposition to drinking water fluoridation has grown, based on the scientific literature documenting the increasingly out-of-control exposures to fluoride, the lack of benefit to dental health from ingestion of fluoride and the hazards to human health from such ingestion. These hazards include acute toxic hazard, such as to people with impaired kidney function, as well as chronic toxic hazards of gene mutations, cancer, reproductive effects, neurotoxicity, bone pathology and dental fluorosis. First, a review of recent neurotoxicity research results.

In 1995, Mullenix and co-workers showed that rats given fluoride in drinking water at levels that give rise to plasma fluoride concentrations in the range seen in humans suffer neurotoxic effects that vary according to when the rats were given the fluoride – as adult animals, as young animals, or through the placenta before birth.[2] Those exposed before birth were born hyperactive and remained so throughout their lives. Those exposed as young or adult animals displayed depressed activity. Then in 1998, Guan and co-workers gave doses similar to those used by the Mullenix research group to try to understand the mechanism(s) underlying the effects seen by the Mullenix group.[3] Guan's group found that several key chemicals in the brain – those that form the membrane of brain cells – were substantially depleted in rats given fluoride, as compared to those who did not get fluoride.

Another 1998 publication by Varner, Jensen and others reported on the brain and kidney damaging effects in rats that were given fluoride in drinking water at the same level deemed 'optimal' by pro-fluoridation groups, namely 1 part per million (1 ppm).[4] Even more pronounced damage was seen in animals that got the fluoride in conjunction with aluminum. These results are especially disturbing because of the low dose level of fluoride that shows the toxic effect in rats – rats are more resistant to fluoride than humans. This latter statement is based on Mullenix's finding that it takes substantially more fluoride in the drinking water of rats than of humans to reach the same fluoride level in plasma. It is the level in plasma that determines how much fluoride is 'seen' by particular tissues in the body. So when rats get 1 ppm in drinking water, their brains and kidneys are exposed to much less fluoride than humans getting 1 ppm, yet they are experiencing toxic effects. Thus we are compelled to consider the likelihood that humans are experiencing damage to their brains and kidneys at the 'optimal' level of 1 ppm.

In support of this concern are results from two epidemiology studies from China,[5,6] that show decreases in IQ in children who get more fluoride than the control groups of children in each study. These decreases are about 5 to 10 IQ points in children aged 8 to 13 years.

Another troubling brain effect has recently surfaced: fluoride's interference with the function of the brain's pineal gland. The pineal gland produces melatonin, which, among other roles, mediates the body's internal clock, doing such things as governing the onset of puberty. Jennifer Luke has shown that fluoride accumulates in the pineal gland and inhibits its production of melatonin.[7] She showed in test animals that this inhibition causes an earlier onset of sexual maturity, an effect reported in humans as well in 1956, as part of the Kingston/Newburgh study, which is discussed below. In fluoridated Newburgh, young girls experienced earlier onset of menstruation (on average, by six months) than girls in non-fluoridated Kingston.[8]

From a risk assessment perspective, all these brain effect data are particularly compelling and disturbing because they are convergent.

We looked at the cancer data with alarm as well. There are epidemiology studies that are convergent with whole-animal and single-cell studies (dealing with the cancer hazard), just as the neurotoxicity research just mentioned all points in the same direction. EPA fired the Office of Drinking Water's chief toxicologist, Dr William Marcus, who also was our local union's treasurer at the time, for refusing to remain silent on the cancer risk issue.[9] The judge who heard the lawsuit he brought against EPA over the firing made that finding – that EPA fired him over his fluoride work and not for the phony reason put forward by EPA management at his dismissal. Dr Marcus won his lawsuit and is again at work at EPA. Documentation is available on request.

The type of cancer of particular concern with fluoride, although not the only type, is osteosarcoma, especially in males. The National Toxicology Program conducted a two-year study in which rats and mice were given sodium fluoride in drinking water.[10] The positive result of that study (in which malignancies in tissues other than bone were also observed), particularly in male rats, is convergent with a host of data from tests showing fluoride's ability to cause mutations (a principal 'trigger' mechanism for inducing a cell to become cancerous)[11] and data showing increases in osteosarcomas in young men in New Jersey,[12] Washington and Iowa[13] based on their drinking fluoridated water. It was his analysis, repeated statements about all these and other incriminating cancer data, and his requests for an independent, unbiased evaluation of them that got Dr Marcus fired.

Bone pathology other than cancer is a concern as well. An excellent review of this issue was published by Diesendorf et al. in 1997.[14] Five epidemiology studies have shown a higher rate of hip fractures in fluoridated vs. non-fluoridated communities.[15] Crippling skeletal fluorosis was the endpoint used by EPA to set its primary drinking water standard in 1986, and the ethical deficiencies in that standard setting process prompted our union to join the Natural Resources Defense Council in opposing the standard in court, as mentioned above.

Regarding the effectiveness of fluoride in reducing dental cavities, there has not been any double-blind study of fluoride's effectiveness as a caries preventative. There have been many, many small scale, selective publications on this issue that proponents cite to justify fluoridation, but the largest and most comprehensive study, one done by dentists trained by the National Institute of Dental Research, on over 39,000 school children aged 5–17 years, shows no significant differences (in terms of decayed, missing and filled teeth) among caries incidences in fluoridated, non-fluoridated and partially fluoridated communities.[16] The latest publication on the fifty-year fluoridation experiment in two New York cities, Newburgh and Kingston, shows the same thing.[17] The only significant difference in dental health between the two communities as a whole is that fluoridated Newburgh, NY, shows about twice the incidence of dental fluorosis (the first, visible sign of fluoride chronic toxicity) as seen in non-fluoridated Kingston.

John Colquhoun's publication on this point of efficacy is especially important.[18] Dr Colquhoun was principal dental officer for Auckland, the largest city in New Zealand, and a staunch supporter of fluoridation – until he was given the task of looking at the world-wide data on fluoridation's effectiveness in preventing cavities. The paper is titled, 'Why I Changed My Mind about Water Fluoridation.' In it Colquhoun provides details on how data were manipulated to support fluoridation in English speaking countries, especially the

US and New Zealand. This paper explains why an ethical public health professional was compelled to do a 180 degree turn on fluoridation.

Further on the point of the tide turning against drinking water fluoridation, statements are now coming from other dentists in the pro-fluoride camp who are starting to warn that topical fluoride (e.g. fluoride in tooth paste) is the only significantly beneficial way in which that substance affects dental health.[19,20,21] However, if the concentrations of fluoride in the oral cavity are sufficient to inhibit bacterial enzymes and cause other bacteriostatic effects, then those concentrations are also capable of producing adverse effects in mammalian tissue, which likewise relies on enzyme systems. This statement is based not only on common sense, but also on results of mutation studies which show that fluoride can cause gene mutations in mammalian and lower order tissues at fluoride concentrations estimated to be present in the mouth from fluoridated tooth paste.[22] Further, there were tumors of the oral cavity seen in the NTP cancer study mentioned above, further strengthening concern over the toxicity of topically applied fluoride.

In any event, a person can choose whether to use fluoridated tooth paste or not (although finding non-fluoridated kinds is getting harder and harder), but one cannot avoid fluoride when it is put into the public water supplies.

So, in addition to our concern over the toxicity of fluoride, we note the uncontrolled – and apparently uncontrollable – exposures to fluoride that are occurring nationwide via drinking water, processed foods, fluoride pesticide residues and dental care products. A recent report in the lay media,[23] that, according to the Centers for Disease Control, at least 22 per cent of America's children now have dental fluorosis, is just one indication of this uncontrolled, excess exposure. The finding of nearly 12 per cent incidence of dental fluorosis among children in unfluoridated Kingston, New York, is another.[17] For governmental and other organizations to continue to push for more exposure in the face of current levels of over-exposure coupled with an increasing crescendo of adverse toxicity findings is irrational and irresponsible at best.

Thus, we took the stand that a policy which makes the public water supply a vehicle for disseminating this toxic and prophylactically useless (via ingestion, at any rate) substance is wrong.

We have also taken a direct step to protect the employees we represent from the risks of drinking fluoridated water. We applied EPA's risk control methodology, the Reference Dose, to the recent neurotoxicity data. The Reference Dose is the daily dose, expressed in milligrams of chemical per kilogram of body weight, that a person can receive over the long term with reasonable assurance of safety from adverse effects. Application of this methodology to the Varner, et al.[14] data leads to a Reference Dose for fluoride of 0.000007 mg/kg-day. Persons who drink about one quart of fluoridated water from the public drinking water supply of the District of Columbia while at work receive about 0.001 mg/kg-day from that source alone. This amount of fluoride is more than 100 times the Reference Dose. On the basis of these results the union filed a grievance, asking that EPA provide unfluoridated drinking water to its employees.

The implication for the general public of these calculations is clear. Recent, peer-reviewed toxicity data, when applied to EPA's standard method for controlling risks from toxic chemicals, require an immediate halt to the use of the nation's drinking water reservoirs as disposal sites for the toxic waste of the phosphate fertilizer industry.[2]

Conclusion

Dr Hirzy's statement on behalf of the EPA scientists speaks for itself. The EPA may back water fluoridation – it is after all a US government agency, and the US government supports fluoridation – but its employees certainly don't.

References

The above statement with references is at http://www.npwa.freeserve.co.uk/epastatement.html.

12. Support for Fluoridation Diminishes in America

Is it true that several American organisations have withdrawn their endorsement of fluoridation?

BFS suggested answer

No. Neither the American Dental Association nor the US Public Health Service is aware of any reputable organisation which has withdrawn its support for fluoridation.

BFS suggested answer refuted

The ACLU has never endorsed or taken any position on the merits of water fluoridation, nor have we ever to my knowledge authorized the American Dental Association to list the ACLU as endorsing the practice.

Ira Glasser, executive director, American Civil Liberties Union, 21 January 1997

In the introduction to this book I listed the organisations that, the British Fluoridation Society claims, endorse and support its stance on the compulsory mass medication that is water fluoridation in Britain. The American Dental Association publishes a similar list. However, some of those listed, like the American Civil Liberties Union, from which I got the above quote, have never supported fluoridation, and others that formerly supported it have had second thoughts. Below is a list of those organisations that have withdrawn their support recently. The BFS, the ADA and US public health service might like to use it to update their lists.

US organisations that have withdrawn their support for fluoridation since 1990:

American Academy of Allergy and Immunology
American Academy of Diabetes
American Cancer Society
American Chiropractic Association
American Civil Liberties Union
American Diabetes Association
American Nurses Association
American Parent–Teachers Association
American Psychiatric Association
Child Study Association of America
Chronic Fatigue Syndrome Activation Network
Commission on Chronic Illness
Federation of American Societies for Experimental Biology
Joint Committee on Health Problems in Education
National Kidney Foundation
National Institute of Municipal Law Officers
Society of Toxicology

The BFS's suggested answer is qualified, as they talk of no 'reputable' organisation withdrawing its support. Perhaps the BFS doesn't consider the organisations listed above to be reputable?

Many North American communities have also rejected fluoridation since 1990. On 7 November 2000, there was a nationwide referendum on fluoridation in the USA's unfluoridated communities. Two-thirds of them voted No. Other referendums in Canada in 2000 also produced votes against fluoridation.[1]

References

1. http://www.fluoridealert.org/e-2000.htm. Accessed 30 December 2000.

13. The Totality of Fluoride

Why do health authorities ignore the World Health Organization warning that they should be aware of total fluoride exposure before introducing fluoridation?

BFS suggested answer

The World Health Organization considers appropriately fluoridated water and routine toothbrushing with a fluoride toothpaste a basic level of protection against tooth decay. The WHO does not recommend that health authorities should be aware of total fluoride exposure before introducing fluoridation.

BFS suggested answer refuted

In the assessment of the safety of a water supply with respect to the fluoride concentration, the total daily fluoride intake by the individual must be considered. *Apart from variations in climatic conditions, it is well known that in certain areas, fluoride-containing foods form an important part of the diet. The facts should be borne in mind in deciding the concentration of fluoride to be permitted in drinking water.*
WHO, 1971 (emphasis added)

The BFS's suggested answer is a vain attempt to sidestep the issue because they *have* ignored the WHO's warning. The word 'recommend' is not used by the WHO, but that was not the question. What the WHO actually said in 1971 is quoted above.[1] And the BFS has ignored it.

The reason we need to be aware of *total* fluoride intakes before even more is added is that fluoride levels have been rising over the past half-century. As we saw in Chapter 4, fluoride intakes from a wide range of sources have increased dramatically since fluoridation was introduced half a century ago.

An uncontrolled experiment

In 1997 I decided to do an experiment. I do not use a fluoridated toothpaste, I eat very little that comes in a packet or tin, I don't use non-stick cookware (another significant source of fluoride), I had stopped drinking tea, and the tap water in my area contains only 0.13 ppm of naturally occurring calcium fluoride. In that year I sent a sample of my urine to a laboratory for analysis. I had expected that it would show a negligible fluoride intake. However, I was horrified to discover, when the results came back, that they indicated I had an intake of 1.5 mg per day. Thus, I am consuming 50 per cent more than is 'needed to protect my teeth', and half the safe amount – and I am actively trying to avoid it altogether!

Conclusion

Over the half-century that fluoridation has been practised, fluoride intakes have risen alarmingly. Just how much fluoride are people taking in? Estimates in the 1950s put total intake at less than 1 mg per day; latest figures say it is approaching 8 mg. The UK Department of Health estimates that the average daily consumption in fluoridated areas in Britain is 2.9 mg per day. But this estimate is merely a guess, and not even an educated guess at that, because the Department of Health has never actually measured fluoride intakes – so it simply doesn't know what the real intake is. The WHO warning needs to be taken seriously.

References

1. WHO. *International drinking water standards.* World Health Organization, 1971.

14. The Ethics and Legality of Fluoridation

Why should everyone be forced to ingest fluoride in their water whether they want to or not. Surely those people who want fluoride can use fluoride toothpaste or tablets?

BFS suggested answer
All water contains some fluoride. Water supplies in some areas, such as Hartlepool, naturally contain just the right amount, and tooth decay rates there are very low. Elsewhere, in Birmingham and Newcastle for example, the natural level is topped up and greatly benefits everyone in terms of better dental health for both young and old.

Drinking fluoride-free water is not a basic human right but a question of individual preference. In society individual preferences must be balanced against the common good.

BFS suggested answer refuted
The debate should not be the merits of fluoridation of the water supply, which is a public health problem, but rather the ethical aspects of universal fluoridation, which creates an untenable situation for those individuals who are intolerant to fluorides. Do we have the moral right to create a situation from which the intolerant individual has no escape? The answer thus becomes very simple. Each individual should be granted the option to choose fluoride prophylaxis depending upon his need and tolerance.
Ben F. Feingold, MD

Fluoridation is bad medicine

Fluoridation is often likened by its proponents to vaccination of children against contagious diseases. Such vaccinations are seldom contested, as it is generally recognised that where diseases are communicable or highly contagious in a public setting, they may lead to a general epidemic. This is the basis for the BFS's answer.

But dental caries is neither communicable nor contagious. There is therefore no substantial threat to the general public health and safety. Those citizens most susceptible to this non-communicable disease can seek treatment individually by more discretely targeted means; there is no need to mass medicate the entire citizenry.

The protection of teeth by fluoridation is merely attempting to mitigate the symptoms of disease without first trying to cure the disease. This is not good medicine. If dentists are really concerned about dental caries, why are they not openly addressing the cause: children's eating of sweets, fizzy drinks and other refined carbohydrates (starches and sugars)?

One of the things on which both sides of the fluoridation debate agree is that too much fluoride can be harmful. It matters not, therefore, whether it is good for teeth or whether it is safe at the correct dosage: if that dosage is uncontrolled, as it is in drinking water, it is possible for people to take an overdose. Proponents will argue that 1 ppm is a controlled dose, but this is a false argument. People drink different amounts of water, depending on the weather or their health or their liking for water. This, surely, must be self-evident, and claims to the contrary cannot be soundly based. Dr Peter Mansfield, director of the Templegarth Trust in the UK, summed up the position well when he said:

> No physician in his right senses would prescribe for a person he has never met, whose medical history he does not know, a substance which is intended to create bodily

change, with the advice: 'Take as much as you like, but you will take it for the rest of your life because some children suffer from tooth decay.' It is a preposterous notion.

Fluoridation is tyranny

Fluoridation is an affront to human dignity, which is explicitly recognised as a major objective in the United Nations Declaration of Human Rights. The foundation of the legal rights and liberties of the individual is the principle of that individual's responsibility for his conduct and his own interests, chief among which is his health.

Many people believe that in a democracy, if a majority can be persuaded to vote in favour of doing something, then that thing should be done. This belief is a perverse and false view of democracy. The principles of democracy, as enshrined in the UN Declaration, are primarily concerned with the rights of people as individuals, *not* with dominance by the majority. If 51 per cent of an electorate vote for medication for the entire population, they are denying the other 49 per cent their basic human rights. This is not democracy but tyranny.

If we wish to ensure the survival of democracy in Britain, Ireland and elsewhere, all of us, collectively and as individuals, have a responsibility to ensure that its principles are not undermined. We can enjoy the full benefits of democracy only if we play our individual parts in protecting those rights, both for ourselves and for each other.

In the Anglo-American democratic system of government, members of parliament and local councillors act as our representatives. As such, they have responsibilities to those who elected them. Their primary duty is to protect the basic rights of the individual citizen from possible tyranny by a misled and thoughtless majority. Compulsory fluoridation automatically violates these rights. Thus, whatever individual

MPs (or in Ireland, TDs) or local councillors believe about the benefits or otherwise of fluoridation, it is their manifest duty to reject proposals to fluoridate the water.

In the UK, although elected members of parliament enact the laws that permit fluoridation, and elected local councillors are consulted about fluoridation in their areas, it is currently the members of area health authorities who decide whether a particular area shall be fluoridated – and they are not elected. Thus, they can never even claim that they have a democratic right to do such a thing.

Is fluoridation unlawful?

In the UK, Ireland and many other countries, it is a fundamental legal principle that no doctor may prescribe medical treatment for a sane and competent person without that person's consent, even if that person is the doctor's own patient and the doctor knows the patient's medical history and medical needs. In view of this law, how can it be right, lawful or ethical for health authorities to prescribe medication for persons they have not met, whose past medical histories and medical needs they do not know, where the dose that each individual will take is neither known nor controlled, when it is not known whether the medication will react with other medications being taken, or even whether those persons need the medication at all?

When a medicine is not a medicine

The argument that people have a right not to be medicated without their consent has always been countered by the pro-fluoridationist riposte that fluoridation is not medication.

I wrote to the Medicines Control Agency (MCA) about this. David Carter, Borderline Section manager, Inspection and Enforcement Division, replied that:

> One of the duties of the Medicines Control Agency (MCA) is to determine whether or not a product is a medicine as defined in Article 1 of Directive 65/65/EEC. It is the considered view that fluoridated drinking water is not a medicine within that definition. Accordingly fluoridated water is not subject to the controls of the Medicines for Human Use (Marketing Authorisations Etc.) Regulations 1994 (as amended) or the Medicines Act 1968 and subsidiary legislation.

The definition in Article 1 of Directive 65/65/EEC he referred to is:

2. Medicinal product: Any substance or combination of substances presented for treating or preventing disease in human beings or animals.

3. Substance: Any matter, irrespective of origin, which may be:– chemical, e.g. elements, naturally occurring chemical materials and chemical products obtained by chemical change or synthesis.[1]

That seems clear and unambiguous. Dental caries is a disease in which a part of the body – the teeth – is damaged by bacterial infection. The sole object of fluoridation is:

1. The prevention of this damage by the strengthening of dental enamel;

2. Its treatment by the killing of the bacteria.

Thus, fluoridation must surely, by the definition above, be a 'medicinal product'. I can see no other interpretation. So why doesn't the MCA consider fluoridated water to be a medicine?

I wrote to the MCA again.

This time Mr Carter wrote back: '[T]he MCA has determined that the inclusion of fluoride in the water supply, *in the concentration in which it is included*, does not make that supply a licensable medicinal product within Directive

65/65/EEC.' (Emphasis in the original)

This despite the facts that fluoride has been used to treat Graves' disease (overactive thyroid)[2] since 1926 at concentrations *lower* than the 1 mg per litre put in drinking water,[3] and that *underactive* thyroid is treated with doses of thyroxine of the order of micrograms.[4]

Mr Carter also wrote that Britain and other EC member states consider that 'such a water supply is not a substance or combination of substances "presented for treating or preventing disease in human beings"'.

I fail to understand why putting fluoride in the water to treat and prevent dental caries is not 'treating or preventing disease in human beings'.

Am I missing something?

Is fluoridation contrary to the European Convention on Human Rights?

The Council of Europe's Convention for the Protection of Human Rights and Dignity of the Human Being with regard to the Application of Biology and Medicine: Convention on Human Rights and Biomedicine, which came into force on 2 October 2000, defines the medical ethics that apply to the contamination of the public water supply with any substance – regardless of motive.

Water fluoridation is clearly an infringement of Article 1, which states: '**Parties to this Convention shall . . . guarantee everyone . . . respect for their integrity and other rights and fundamental freedoms with regard to the application of biology and medicine.**' This means that anyone who objects to taking a medication has the right to refuse consent and avoid exposure for both themselves and their family.

Article 2 states: '**The interests and welfare of the human being shall prevail over the sole interest of the society or science.**' This clearly establishes that where there is a conflict of interests, the interests of the individual override those of the State. The current policy, that health authorities and water companies should decide whether fluoride is to be fed to the public at large in the face of objections, is clearly in breach of this.

Article 5 states: '**An intervention in the health field may only be carried out after the person concerned has given free and informed consent to it.**' Water fluoridation has never been introduced with the consent of all the people. It requires only one person to withhold his or her permission for the imposition of water fluoridation to be unethical under the provisions of the Convention, and by association, under any code of medical ethics. This article also requires that: '**This person shall beforehand be given appropriate information as to the purpose and nature of the intervention as well as on its consequences and risks.**' If the government decides that drinking water is to be fluoridated, every single person within the area to be fluoridated should receive a full, easily understood, balanced and accurate statement of both the advantages *and the disadvantages* of fluoridation. This must be accompanied by a full risk analysis for a lifetime's exposure, supported by clear indications of where and how any member of the population could verify that the literature presented was scientifically correct and unbiassed, and that adequate safeguards were in place to protect their interests. Finally, Article 5 states: '**The person concerned may freely withdraw consent at any time.**' Thus, if any person says he or she no longer wishes to be fluoridated, fluoridation must cease for that person.

The European Convention as it applies to Britain and Ireland

The European Convention, which is now accepted as a reasonable representative framework of public and medical ethics for dealing with medical interventions, was incorporated into the UK's new Human Rights Act, which also came into force on 2 October 2000. It applies to medical interventions practised both at the individual level and on populations. It requires signatories to establish legislation that includes legal sanctions, and it requires compensation for individuals who have suffered undue damages following any medical treatment or research.

Although the British government is not a signatory to the whole of this Convention, the European Court has ruled that what may once have been an allowable restriction of private rights may not be allowable now, and that courts are now required to interpret the new Civil Procedure Rules in ways that are compatible with the European Convention, and not necessarily with the British interpretation of it.

Action against public authorities and individuals

Under the Human Rights Act in the UK, action can be taken only against 'public authorities'. Under the terms of the Act:

- All suppliers of services to the public are considered to be 'public authorities': national government, local councils, schools, NHS hospitals, water supply companies, regulatory bodies such as Offwat, public advice services, and the courts. Water companies have an obvious risk under the new Act.

- The Act also applies to any individual whose functions are 'of a public nature'. Thus, dentists and BFS members who advocate fluoridation, and who do so while being funded by government, will be individually liable for damages should their advice result in damage to any person – a position that carries serious potential financial risk.

- Food manufacturers and packers will also have to be careful not to use water that may contain fluoride added improperly by a public authority. Although in this case, whether the consumer would bring an action against the water supplier or the food manufacturer could exercise legal minds.

- Article 3 requires the State to prevent breaches of the Act by one private individual against another and to prevent violations of rights by private persons – this would apply to corporate entities as well as individual persons. Any exclusion incorporated in new British legislation with the purpose of allowing such compulsory medication as fluoridation, therefore, may well be seen as a breach of the European Convention – and European legislation takes precedent.

The European Charter of Fundamental Rights

While paying lip service to the new Human Rights Act, the British government has not signed up to all its conventions. In so doing, the government believes it can override the law as it applies to fluoridation in England and Wales (the law in Scotland is different), as such laws as the Water (Fluoridation) Act can be retained even though they are clearly contrary to medical ethics.

But on the horizon looms another draft act, the European Charter of Fundamental Rights, which challenges this unilateral declaration of exemption for England. The British government has endorsed this draft act. When it comes into force, any British legislation, such as compulsory medication without consent, that permits the State to violate the rights of the people will be in violation of the European Convention. The situation at present is that the new Human Rights Act as it applies to fluoridation must be tested in the courts. When the Charter comes onto the statute books, that will spell the end of fluoridation in this country, in Ireland and in any other member country of the EU.

Medical experimentation

On 21 February 2001, *The Independent* reported that children at a dozen nursery and infant schools in South Yorkshire were to be given 'dental milk' which had been treated with fluoride.

This was mentioned at the end of Chapter 6 as an example of the lack of knowledge displayed by the BFS. But there is another side to this story — a human rights dimension. The plan is to have specially labelled bottles of fluoridated milk, which will be provided only to children whose parents have given written consent. Herein lies the first legal problem.

Dr John Rental, the British Dental Association's chairman warned in the article of possible legal action from parents of children given treated milk by mistake. 'The issue of public health measures is always loaded with problems about consent, safety and liability,' he said. 'With fluoride, there is an issue if a parent has not given consent and then their child drinks another's fluoride milk.' Sue King of the North and Midlands Against Fluoridation campaign group wants to know how teachers are going to monitor this.

The second legal problem is that, as the BFS cannot have definitive proof of the efficacy and safety of this measure, what they are initiating is an uncontrolled experiment using infants as the guinea pigs. That opens up a whole new field of potential litigation.

Conclusion

Fluoridation as it is now practised has many ethical and legal implications. Health authorities, local councils and their individual members may be liable under the Human Rights Act if they support fluoridation, since the practice clearly violates both medical ethics and human rights. The Act is particularly concerned that the rights of children – the very people at whom fluoridation is aimed – should be protected.

Thus, education departments will be in breach of the Act if they permit the use of fluoridated water or milk in schools.

The impact of the new Human Rights Act and the forthcoming European Charter of Fundamental Rights is likely to be far wider than many people realise. It is ironic that the Act states that the State is legally responsible for protecting the rights of the individual – when it is the State that is in violation of the Act in its promotion of fluoridation. Our rulers and decision-makers should consider very carefully the fact that failure of British government bodies to conform to the Convention's standard of ethics may place them in a very precarious legal position.

References

1. 365L0065. Council Directive 65/65/EEC, 26 January 1965, on the approximation of provisions laid down by Law, Regulation or Administrative Action relating to proprietary medicinal products. Chapter I: Definitions and scope, Article 1. This may be accessed at http://europa.eu.int/eur-lex/en/lif/dat/1965/en_365L0065.html.

2. Goldemberg L. Action physiologique des fluorures. *Compt Rend Soc Physiol* (Paris) 1926; 95: 1169.

3. von Mundy G. Einfluss von Fluor und Jod auf den Stoffwechsel, insbesondere auf die Schilddrüse. *Münch Med Wochenschrift* 1963; 105: 234–47.

4. *Monthly index of medical specialities* (MIMS). London: Haymarket Publishing Services, 2001.

15. Dental Fluorosis

Is it true that up to 80 per cent of children living in fluoridated areas suffer from dental fluorosis?

BFS suggested answer

No. In the UK unsightly dental fluorosis is rare. However, tooth decay is a huge problem which affects millions of children. Ugly black holes in children's teeth caused by decay are the ugliest problem of all.

BFS suggested answer refuted

Dental fluorosis, no matter how slight, is an irreversible pathological condition recognised by authorities around the world as the first readily detectable clinical symptom of previous chronic fluoride poisoning. To suggest we should ignore such a sign is as irrational as saying that the blue-black line which appears on the gums due to chronic lead poisoning is of no significance because it doesn't cause any pain or discomfort.
Dr Geoffrey Smith[1]

There are many disorders, considered in other chapters, that those opposed to fluoridation claim are caused by fluoride and that those in favour of fluoridation refuse to accept are related to it. But there is one very obvious condition caused by fluoride that is not disputed. That is the staining or mottling of teeth called dental fluorosis.

While there is agreement on both sides that fluorosis exists, and that fluorosis is an undesirable side effect of fluoride use, the two sides differ in their attitudes to it. Those in favour of fluoride say that fluorosis is 'a cosmetic issue, not a health problem';[2] that in its mildest form the pearly-white patches of fluorosis actually make teeth 'more attractive than teeth without fluorosis'.[3] Anti-fluoridationists take a different view: that fluorosis is a visible sign of fluoride poisoning.

Who is right?

Dental fluorosis was first reported by two dentists in 1916.[4] By 1931, there was extreme concern about what was called 'Colorado brown stain' and 'Texas teeth'. In that year three independent groups of scientists[5,6,7] showed conclusively that the areas with this condition had high levels of fluoride in their water.

Reports from China,[8] Argentina,[9] Britain,[10] Italy[11] and Japan[12] also showed significant levels of fluorosis in children drinking fluoride-contaminated water. Many of these reports were from areas with levels of fluoride in their water of the order of 8 or more parts per million. But then it was noticed that fluorosis was not restricted to areas with such high levels. In a 1982 study carried out by the University of Rochester, USA, fluorosis was seen in 28 per cent of children aged between eleven and thirteen, yet they were drinking water with the recommended level of 1 ppm.[13] Later studies showed a similar picture across North America, with an average fluorosis in the school population of 40.5 per cent,[14] while it was as high as 58 per cent in Quebec,[15] and 69.2 per cent in Nova Scotia.[16] Researchers in the Netherlands reported that 74 per cent of children examined exhibited fluorosis in a slight to moderate degree.[17] They say that more teeth were affected and the degree of mottling was higher when children started to use fluoride at an earlier age. By 1989, over 80 per cent of 12- to 14-year-old children in Augusta, Georgia, had fluorosis.[18]

Dental fluorosis also affects a large proportion of children in the fluoridated areas of Britain.[19] It is particularly easy to spot in large fluoridated cities like Birmingham, where the vast majority of children seem to suffer from it.

With the coming of fluoridated toothpastes, infant formulas, and commercially prepared beverages – in particular, soft drinks such as colas – made with fluoridated water, the incidence of dental fluorosis has increased, even in unfluoridated areas.

There are regular warnings in the dental press, such as: 'Dentists should be aware of the fluoride concentrations of the drinking water of their child patients, be they municipal or bottled drinking water, when prescribing fluoride supplements,' or 'Practitioners should estimate fluoride ingestion from all these sources if considering systemic fluoride supplementation.' But how can dentists – or anyone else – make any form of meaningful estimation when no official body measures individual intakes of fluoride?

It took fifty years, after the first fluoridation scheme was introduced, for the American Dental Association to acknowledge that fluorosis was a problem. 'This has led to efforts to identify the cause or causes,' they say.[20] But we all know what the cause is: it's no secret, we've known it for almost a century – it's fluoride! The author suggested that dental practitioners could have an important impact on reducing the prevalence of enamel fluorosis by guiding the public toward the most appropriate use of fluoride products. Of course they could. The question is: Why don't they?

Breast is best

A major source of fluoride in infancy is infant formulas. Whether or not they are made with fluoridated water, infant formulas have been implicated as a risk factor for fluorosis in several studies. Doctors in Melbourne, Australia, found that the fluoride content of commonly used infant formulas in Australia ranged from 0.23 to 3.71 ppm if the formulas were milk-based and from 1.08 to 2.86 ppm if they were soy-based.[21] When the formulas were reconstituted, according to the manufacturer's directions, with fluoridated water, infants' intakes were as much as three times the recommended upper limit.

On the other hand, breast milk contains very little fluoride. Because fluorine is such a ubiquitous element, practically everything we eat or drink contains some fluoride. During our evolution we must have developed a tolerance for small quantities of it. But no matter how much is found in the foods and water a mother drinks, it seems to be filtered out in some way, for very little, 0.01 ppm on average, is found in breast milk.[22] This indicates that nature has designed things so that infants are protected from fluorides in their early years.

Fluoride supplements

For areas that do not have the 'benefit' of fluoridated water, parents have been persuaded to give their offspring fluoride pills, drops or similar supplements. The effects of such supplementation on dental caries and dental fluorosis was measured in 160 children in two age ranges: 7–9 years and 11–14 years. They all had lived from birth in a region with low fluoride levels in the drinking water, and had been offered sodium fluoride supplementation in the form of drops for daily use. Inevitably some children complied with the recommendations religiously, while others didn't. The results showed no statistically significant differences in dental caries between the regular and irregular users of fluoride supplementation. Considerable dental fluorosis was found in 38–63 per cent of the children in both groups.[23]

There have been many calls for the use of fluoride supplements to cease. In 1991 the US government published its estimated intake of fluoride for Americans, which was as much as 120 per cent over the assigned 'optimal dose' of 1 mg per day in unfluoridated areas and a huge 605 per cent in fluoridated areas. The government said that its data indicated that dentists should not prescribe supplements.[24] The Canadian Dental Association recommends 'No fluoride supplements for children under seven years old'.

It seems that this entreaty was unsuccessful, as subsequently there have been more calls for the cessation of fluoride supplementation. In 1994 Dr Brian Burt of Ann Arbor, Michigan, told the Dietary Fluoride Supplement Conference of the American Dental Association, in Chicago, Illinois, that there are three reasons why the use of supplements was inappropriate among young children in the United States:[25]

- The evidence for the efficacy of fluoride supplements in caries prevention was not strong.

- Supplements were a clear risk for dental fluorosis.

- Fluoride did not protect teeth that had yet to appear.

The last reason is particularly relevant to water fluoridation. The proponents of fluoride say that it has its greatest effects while teeth are growing. Indeed, after teeth have grown and matured, fluoride cannot be incorporated. Bones in the body are dynamic structures in that their materials are constantly being replaced. For that reason, fluoride is incorporated throughout life. This is not the case with teeth. Once they have grown and matured, they are static. After about the age of twelve, therefore, only a topical application – toothpaste, gels, and so on – can direct fluoride to where it may do any good.

Calls for supplementation to cease were not confined to America. In 1996 Dr P.J. Riordan, of Western Australia, pointed to the substantial evidence that supplements caused dental fluorosis even when used in accordance with recommendations for infants and small children.[26] He warned:

Supplements should no longer be recommended for caries prevention in children in areas with little fluoride in water . . . If supplements are recommended for children, a more cautious dosage schedule should be used. The fact that supplements have been recommended uncritically for many years on the basis of inadequate research raises questions about the standards of dental science.

It is clear that any benefit from supplement use is marginal at best, while the risk of fluorosis is high. Dr Burt stated that '[t]here is evidence that the public is more aware of the milder forms of fluorosis than was previously thought, so dental policies should be aimed at reducing fluorosis'. I am disturbed by the reason Burt gives – that the public is more aware of fluorosis. Shouldn't health be the main criterion? He continued: 'The risks of using fluoride supplements in young children outweigh the benefits. Since there are alternative forms of fluoride to use in high-risk individuals, fluoride supplements should no longer be used for young children in North America.'

Toothpaste

Systemic use of fluoride from water, food and supplements has not been shown to have a statistical benefit in terms of reduction of caries but has merely led to a dramatic increase in fluorosis. What evidence there is suggests that a topical application of fluoride directly to the tooth's surface may be more effective at combatting decay. But does this also increase the risk of fluorosis? Dr M.C. Skotowski and colleagues set out to answer this question in Iowa City in 1995. A total of 157 children aged eight to seventeen, who sought dental treatment in a university paediatric dental clinic, were examined for dental fluorosis. The children's parents were asked to complete fluoride history questionnaires to assess exposure to fluoride during the first eight years of life. Finding fluorosis in 72 per cent of the children, they concluded that '[t]his study provided evidence that increased use of fluoride toothpaste may be a risk factor for dental fluorosis. The results suggest prudent use of dentifrice by young children to minimise the risk of fluorosis.'[27]

How much fluoride does it take to cause fluorosis?

The answer seems to be: very little. The recommended 'optimal' level of 1 ppm has been shown time and time again to cause fluorosis. There is no doubt about this; even the pro-fluoridationists admit that fluorosis can occur at this level.

But does it matter?

Dentists say that fluorosis is merely a minor cosmetic condition. But it is not 'minor' if you happen to suffer from it. Fluorosis strikes when a child is at a psychologically vulnerable age. Children with badly stained (fluorosed) teeth tend to be shunned, bullied or ridiculed by their peers. No child should have to endure that. At an international conference on fluoridation in Birmingham in 1995, evidence was presented that 'even mild [fluorosis] was associated with psycho-behavioural impacts'.[28]

It would be bad enough if the harm that fluorosis does stopped at mere childhood intolerance, but it doesn't. Dental fluorosis is not merely a stain on teeth: it is a visible sign of damage to bones and other tissues throughout the body – damage that cannot be seen.[29]

Ingested fluoride is absorbed mainly through the stomach and intestine into the bloodstream. The fluoride is then carried to developing tooth buds, where the fluoride is incorporated into a tooth's enamel. Once there, interaction with the developing crystals initiates the replacement of the tooth enamel's normal crystalline composition, hydroxy-apatite, by fluorapatite, a related crystal that incorporates the fluoride, thus changing the tooth's chemical structure. As fluorapatite is more resistant to decay than hydroxyapatite, this modification of the tooth's chemistry is believed to lead to a reduction in dental caries.

But while fluorapatite may be harder and more resistant to decay, it makes the tooth's enamel more brittle. As fluorosis increases, the subsurface enamel all along the tooth becomes increasingly porous (hypomineralised), leading to extensive mechanical breakdown of the surface.[30] Even with very mild fluorosis, the brittleness makes dental work more difficult and more expensive – a particularly important consideration in undernourished children, who are at a much higher risk of developing dental fluorosis, as their parents are less likely to be able to afford the sometimes expensive cosmetic repairs needed.

The American Dental Association reported that dentists make 17 per cent more profit in fluoridated areas than in unfluoridated areas.[31] This finds support in fluoridated Birmingham, England: although the population has remained fairly constant over the past few decades, the number of dentists practising there doubled over a twenty-year period.

Conclusion

Proponents of water fluoridation admit that those who drink water containing fluoride will suffer fluorosis of their teeth. The only difference between the pro- and anti-fluoride camps is the significance they attach to this fact.

Dental fluorosis is a permanent disfigurement. That is undisputed. Unfortunately for those affected by dental fluorosis, the official position is that their unsightly condition is considered to be merely cosmetic and not an adverse health effect. For this reason, in Britain, for example, treatment cannot be obtained free on the NHS, which seems churlish, when it was the health authorities that caused the problem in the first place.

References

1. Smith G. *New Scientist*, British Fluoridation Society, 5 May 1983.

2. *Dental fluorosis in perspective: The good, the bad and the ugly*. British Fluoridation Society briefing. November 1997.

3. Hawley GM, Ellwood RP, Davis RM. Dental caries, fluorosis and the cosmetic implications of different TF scores in 14-year-old adolescents. *Community Dent Health* 1996; 13: 189–92.

4. Black GV, McKay F. Mottled teeth: An endemic developmental imperfection of the enamel heretofore unknown in the literature of dentistry. *Dent Cosmos* 1916; 58 (2): 129–56.

5. Churchill HV. The occurrence of fluorides in some waters of the United States. *J Am Water Works Assoc* 1931; 23: 1399–403.

6. Smith MC et al. *The cause of mottled enamel, a defect of human teeth*. Technical Bulletin No. 32. University of Arizona College of Agriculture, 10 June 1931.

7. Velu H. Dental dystrophy in mammals of the phosphate zone and chronic fluorosis. *C R Seances Soc Biol Ses Fil* 1931; 108: 750–2.

8. Anderson BG. An endemic center of mottled enamel in China. *J Dent Res* 1932; 12: 591–3.

9. Chaneles J. A dental problem of interest in Argentina: The etiology of 'mottled teeth'. *Rev Odontol* (Buenos Aires) 1932; 20: 64–73.

10. Ainsworth NJ. Mottled teeth. *Br Dent J* 1933; 55: 233–50.

11. Ricci E. The phenomenon of mottled teeth in Italy. *Ann Clin Odontol* 1933; 12: 1029–43.

12. Nakano R. A statistical observation of endemic effects on teeth. *Rinsho Shika* 1933; 2: 102.

13. Leverett D. Fluorides in the changing prevalence of decay rates. *Science* 1982; 217: 26–30.

14. Foulkes RG. Review of 'Investigation of inorganic fluoride and its effect on the occurrence of dental caries and dental fluorosis in Canada – final report'. *Fluoride* 1995; 28: 146–8.

15. Ismail AI, Brodeur JM, Kavanagh M et al. Prevalence of dental caries and dental fluorosis in students, 11–17 years of age, in fluoridated and non-fluoridated cities in Quebec. *Caries Res* 1990; 24: 290–7.

16. Ismail AI, Shoveller J, Langille D, MacInnis WA, McNally M. Should the drinking water of Truro, Nova Scotia, be fluoridated? Water fluoridation in the 1990s. *Community Dent Oral Epidemiol* 1993; 21: 118–25.

17. Woltgens JH, Etty EJ, Nieuwland WM, Lyaruu DM. Use of fluoride by young children and prevalence of mottled enamel. *Adv Dent Res* 1989; 3: 177–82.

18. *Schenectady Gazette Star*, 5 August 1989.

19. Weeks KJ, Milsom KM, Lennon MA. Enamel defects in 4-year-old to 5-year-old children in fluoridated and non-fluoridated parts of Cheshire, UK. *Caries Res* 1993; 27: 317–20.

20. Dendrys D. Risk of fluorosis in a fluoridated population: implications for the dentist and hygienist. *J Am Dent Assoc* 1996; 126: 1617.

21. Silva M, Reynolds EC . Fluoride content of infant formulae in Australia. *Aust Dent J* 1996; 41: 37–42.

22. Levy SM, Kiritsy MC, Warren JJ. Sources of fluoride intake in children. *J Public Health Dent* 1995; 55 (1): 39–52.

23. Awad MA, Hargreaves JA, Thompson GW. Dental caries and fluorosis in 7–9 and 11–14 year old children who received fluoride supplements from birth. *J Can Dent Assoc* 1991; 60: 318–22.

24. *Review of fluoride: Benefits and risks.* US Department of Health and Human Services, 1991; 1–134.

25. Burt BA. *The case for eliminating the use of dietary fluoride supplements among young children.* Abstract of paper presented at Dietary Fluoride Supplement Conference, American Dental Association, Chicago, Illinois, USA, 31 January – 1 February, 1994.

26. Riordan PJ. The place of fluoride supplements in caries prevention today. *Aust Dent J* 1996; 41: 335–42.

27. Skotowski MC, Hunt RJ, Levy SM. Risk factors for dental fluorosis in pediatric dental patients. *J Public Health Dent* 1995; 55: 154–9.

28. Bob Woffinden. Clear and present danger. *The Guardian Weekend* on The Guardian website, www. guardian.co.uk, 7 June 1997.

29. Singh A, Jolly SS. Chronic toxic effects on the skeletal system. In: *Fluorides and human health.* Geneva: WHO, 1970: 238–49.

30. Fejerskov O, Larsen MJ, Richards A, Baelum V. Dental tissue effects of fluoride. *Adv Dent Res* 1994; 8: 15–31.

31. Douglas BL, Wallace DA, Lerner M, Coppersmith SB. Impact of water fluoridation on dental practices and dental manpower. *J Am Dent Assoc* 1972; 84: 355–67.

16. The Dose Makes the Poison

How do you know how much fluoride we are ingesting?

BFS suggested answer
We do not need to know how much fluoride we are ingesting as individuals. There is no evidence that any community in the UK is ingesting too much fluoride.

BFS suggested answer refuted
Investigators seeking to examine the possible relation between fluoride intake and health outcomes, such as dental caries, fluorosis, or quality of bone, need to be aware of the complex situation that exists today. It is no longer feasible to estimate with reasonable accuracy the level of fluoride exposure simply on the basis of concentration in drinking water supply.
US National Research Council, 1993

The US Department of Health and Human Services stated in 1991: 'The total quantity of fluoride ingested is the single most important factor in determining the clinical course of skeletal fluorosis; the severity of symptoms correlates directly with the level and duration of exposure.'' This reiterated the World Health Organization's exhortations for nearly thirty years that the total amount of fluoride must be taken into account before adding yet more.

When fluoridation was first mooted, the amount to be added to water was determined by the belief that 'a person drinking fluoridated water may be assumed to ingest only about 1 milligram per day from this source ... the development of mottled enamel is, however, a potential hazard of adding fluorides to food. The total daily intake of fluoride is the critical quantity.'²

Today, a person's total intake in 'optimally fluoridated' areas is estimated to be between 5 and 7 mg/day. It is not just from water: intake is divided between drinking water (in fluoridated areas), food, other beverages, and dental products. This means that even if you do not live in a fluoridated area, any processed food or drink that is produced outside your area may contain fluoride. Some idea of the widespread nature of the problem is given below:

- Average fluoride content in juices is 0.02–2.80 ppm, in part because of variations in fluoride concentrations in water used in production. Grape juice has been found to contain up to 6.8 mg fluoride per litre, a can of chicken soup up to 4 mg fluoride.

- British toothpastes contain 1,000–1,500 ppm sodium fluoride – you can see the amounts on the packets. Since April 1997, all toothpastes in the USA have carried a poison warning label.

- Fluoride dental treatments can contain between 10,000 and 20,000 ppm fluoride. There is no regulated dose requirement.

- Commercial fresh fruit and vegetables may have been sprayed with a cryolite pesticide.

- Teflon- and Tefal-coated, non-stick cookware releases fluoride into food cooked in them.

The amount of fluoride around today is far greater than it was half a century ago. There is now so much that Dr Hardy Limeback, biochemist and professor of preventive dentistry, University of Toronto, and former consultant to the Canadian Dental Association, said recently: 'Children under three should never use fluoridated toothpaste. Or drink fluoridated water. And baby formula must never be made up using [fluoridated] tap water. Never. In fluoridated areas, people should never use fluoride supplements. We tried to get them banned for children but [the dentists] wouldn't even look at the evidence we presented.'[3]

How much is too much?

All sides agree that healthy kidneys can eliminate only about half of daily fluoride intake. The other half will be retained in the body and will build up over a lifetime in calcified tissues, like bones and teeth. This is what makes it so dangerous.

As little as 0.04 mg/kg body weight per day has been proven to cause adverse health effects. The US National Academy of Sciences stated in 1977 that, for the average individual, a retention of 2 mg/day would result in crippling skeletal fluorosis after forty years. Considering the amount we are ingesting now, it is likely that skeletal fluorosis already affects a significant portion of the population.

Children, the elderly, and any person with impaired kidney function – a category that includes many AIDS and diabetic patients – are in the high-risk group for fluoride poisoning and should be warned to monitor their fluoride intake. Also at high risk are people with immunodeficiencies, diabetes and heart ailments, as well as anyone with calcium, magnesium and Vitamin C deficiencies. At the level of 0.4 ppm fluoride in water, renal (kidney) impairment has been shown.[4]

The BFS is correct that there is a lack of evidence of harm in Britain – but only because no official government or medical authority has ever bothered to look for such evidence. As Professor Susheela said to Mrs Tessa Jowell, British Minister of Health, on 26 October 1998:

> You [the Department of Health] don't even have a government laboratory to test fluoride levels in blood and urine. If you don't look for the problems, how can you hope to find them?[5]

Conclusion

The suggested answer by the BFS is again disingenuous. It shows a contempt for WHO and Department of Health guidelines and warnings.

References

1. *Review of fluoride: Benefits and risks.* US Department of Health and Human Services, February 1991: 45.
2. *The problem of providing optimum fluoride intake for prevention of dental caries.* Food and Nutrition Board, Division of Biology and Agriculture. Publication No. 294, National Academy of Sciences/US National Research Council, November 1953.
3. Limeback H. *Sunday Star*, Toronto, 25 April 1999.
4. Juncos LI, Donadio JV. Renal failure and fluorosis, fluorine and dental health. *J Am Med Assoc* 1972; 222 (7): 783–5.
5. Susheela AK. *Fluoridation of water.* Meeting between Prof. Susheela and Tess Jowek at Richmond House, London, 26 October 1998, arranged by NPWA. Quote published in *Fluoride Watershed*, vol. 4, no. 3, November 1998 by NPWA.

17. Fluoride-Related Bone Problems, Part One

Dr Mansfield of the National Pure Water Association claims that in a few years time we will see an explosion of fluoride-related bone problems in artificially fluoridated areas, but that he is not being taken seriously by the NHS. How do you know that he is wrong if nobody is looking into his claims?

BFS suggested answer

Firstly Dr Mansfield's claims rely on his other claim that there is a difference between artificial and natural fluoridation. There is no difference. Secondly, his work on fluoride intakes in the West Midlands has been reviewed by public health experts in the West Midlands and at the Department of Health, and has been found to be seriously flawed.

Experts at the MRC Environmental Epidemiology Unit conclude that 'the burden of evidence suggesting that fluoridation might be a risk factor for hip fracture is weak and not sufficient to retard the progress of the water fluoridation programme'.

Furthermore, large epidemiological surveys of radiographs in the British population show no evidence of skeletal fluorosis, and neither the early nor late stages of skeletal fluorosis are seen in areas with fluoride at 1 ppm. Nor is there any evidence that other skeletal problems such as stiffness, pain in the joints, backache or osteoarthritis are associated with water fluoridation.

BFS suggested answer refuted

We do know that the use of drinking water containing as little as 1.2–3.0 parts per million of fluorine will cause such developmental disturbances in bones as osteosclerosis, spondylosis and osteopetrosis, as well as goiter, and we cannot afford to run the risk of producing such serious systemic disturbances in applying what is at present a doubtful procedure intended to prevent development of dental disfigurements.
Editorial, *Journal of the American Dental Association*, October 1944

Clearly, fluoride is not as benign a substance as those who promote its use would have us believe. As the quotation from the *Journal of the American Dental Association* above shows, dentists are aware of the dangers at levels above 1.2 ppm. But is it dangerous if our intakes are restricted to the 'optimal' dose of 1.0 ppm or only dangerous if taken to excess? Not that we know how much fluoride is an 'excess' (see Chapter 4), and not that 1.2 ppm is significantly different from 1.0 ppm.

Little research has been conducted into harmful effects of fluoride in Britain and Ireland. Research of this nature is expensive. Normally, only large organisations, such as universities, or bodies funded by industry, can afford to undertake the large and extensive studies needed to achieve statistical significance. But none of them is doing this.

Dr Peter Mansfield, a Lincolnshire GP, director of the Templegarth Trust and, until July 2000, president of the National Pure Water Association, was surprised to discover in 1983 that one of his patients, a girl then aged five years, had 'ailed dramatically' on two occasions, two years apart, when using fluoridated toothpaste. As she recovered promptly when the toothpaste was withdrawn, he came to the conclusion that the girl had been poisoned by the fluoride. Dr Mansfield could find no NHS clinical test for fluoride to help him confirm his diagnosis. He also became concerned at the complete lack of confirmatory evidence of the benefits of fluoride and at the growing incidence of fluorosis, particularly in fluoridated areas. After some preliminary enquiries, he set up his own laboratory facility and began routinely testing for fluoride in 1990.

Mansfield's tests with his patients for fluoride built up a database of more than 700 people living in fluoridated and unfluoridated areas of the East Midlands. Disturbed by his findings on these *unfluoridated* patients, he advertised free fluoride tests in the *Birmingham Evening Mail*, asking for people in the 'flagships of fluoridation' – Coventry, Birmingham and Wolverhampton – to send him samples of their urine for analysis. He initially had replies from 225 people, which, under the circumstances, was a terrific response. Analysis of the samples showed that 57 per cent were ingesting higher than safe levels of fluoride[1] and that the average daily fluoride consumption was more than 4 mg – around 50 per cent higher than government estimates – and in some cases was as high as 17 mg![2] This is nearly six times the government's estimate.

In co-operation with a Coventry osteoporosis support group, Mansfield then checked people with a medical diagnosis of osteoporosis and compared their results with other people from the West Midlands of the same age and sex and with no known medical problems. He discovered that those with osteoporosis consumed nearly twice as much fluoride – an average of 6.3 mg per day, compared with 3.4 mg per day for those who were symptom-free. Mansfield says: 'This substantiates our fear, that a high daily fluoride intake, based on artificially fluoridated water, causes bone disease well before old age – unacceptable if confirmed.'[3]

Knowing the amounts of fluoride that have been proven to cause skeletal fluorosis within an average lifetime, based on Roholm's calculations[4] and Hodge's corrected figures,[5] Dr Mansfield has frequently warned the government of the dangers inherent in water fluoridation. His claims have a solid scientific background and deserve to be taken seriously.

The problem for government, of course, is that if it admits that fluoride is as toxic as we know it is, and if government agencies are found to have known about this all along, it could open the door to compensation claims of such magnitude that the financial stability of the NHS would be threatened. Thus, the government simply dare not do anything that might uncover the truth. But this attitude itself could have serious implications: the more government officials are shown the evidence of harm in interviews such as that between Mrs Tessa Jowell and Professor Susheela in 1998, and the longer the government goes on ignoring them, the greater the likelihood that compensation claims will be successful in the courts.

References

1. Fluoridistas stunned by fluoride lab findings. *Fluoride Watershed*. National Pure Water Association, Crigglestone, South Yorkshire, March 1998.
2. Mansfield P. *We underestimate the damage done by fluorides*. 1997.
3. Mansfield P. *Fresh evidence: Fluoride does damage bones!* Press release, Louth, Lincolnshire, 5 May 1998.
4. Roholm K. *Fluorine intoxication: A clinical–hygienic study*. Copenhagen: Nyt Nordisk, and London: HK Lewis, 1937: 281–2.
5. Hodge HC. *The safety of fluoride tablets or drops in Continuing Evaluation of the Use of Fluorides*. American Association for the Advancement of Science, Westview Press, Boulder, CO, USA, 1979.

18. Fluoride-Related Bone Problems, Part Two

Why does the UK Department of Health refuse to carry out research into Dr Mansfield's claims?

BFS suggested answer

Firstly, it would be irresponsible and unethical to spend public money on a research programme at the whim of one person. The Department of Health continuously monitor all relevant scientific developments relating to fluoridation, and to date there is no evidence at all to support Dr Mansfield's claims.

Secondly, Dr Mansfield's theory is based on the false premise that the fluoride added to the water is not the same as that which occurs naturally. Fluoride ions in solution in water are identical whether they occur naturally in the water or are added.

BFS suggested answer refuted

Based on data from the National Academy of Sciences, current levels of fluoride exposure in drinking water may cause arthritis in a substantial portion of the population long before they reach old age.
Robert J. Carton, PhD, former EPA scientist

The BFS is right to say that the government should not spend taxpayers' money on an expensive research programme at 'the whim of one person'. But that is not the case here. Dr Mansfield is not a lone voice, as the BFS question implies; he represents a large body of scientific opinion. In calling for some proof that fluoride is beneficial and does no harm, he is voicing the concerns of many people not only in Britain but around the world.

The rest of the BFS's suggested answer is quite erroneous. The Department of Health clearly *does not* continuously monitor all relevant scientific developments relating to fluoridation – if it did, it would not be advocating the addition of fluoride to tap water. As to the assertion that 'to date there is no evidence at all to support Dr Mansfield's claims', it must be abundantly obvious that there is a great deal of support for his claims. The reason the Department of Health has no evidence is that it is not looking for it.

And the BFS's other assertion that 'Dr Mansfield's theory is based on the false premise that the fluoride added to the water is not the same as that which occurs naturally', demonstrates either naivety or duplicity – or perhaps it merely confirms the suggested answer in Chapter 6 that its members are not 'experts' in this field and are not competent to deal with this subject. If this really is their interpretation of the science behind fluoridation, one can only agree with that self-appraisal.

19. The Death of Science

Why is it that some doctors and dentists oppose fluoridation?

BFS suggested answer
Organisations representing the medical and dental professions in the UK including the British Dental Association, British Medical Association, and the Royal College of Physicians, and similar organisations worldwide, endorse the safety and efficacy of fluoridation. Those *individuals* who do not support fluoridation are out of step with the views of their professions as a whole. It would be unusual if 100% of any profession agreed on an issue.

BFS suggested answer refuted
Professionalism is about expert judgement, and judgements are apt to differ. On one subject, however, the medical and dental professions in this country have been unanimous for four decades: the benefits and safety of fluoridating drinking water supplies at one part per million.
Dr Peter Mansfield, 1997

Prior to my hearing this case, I gave the matter of fluoridation little if any thought but I received quite an education, and noted that the proponents of fluoridation do nothing more than try to impugn the objectivity of those who oppose fluoridation.
Pennsylvania Supreme Court Justice J.P. Flaherty

Medicine – and that includes dentistry – is as much an art as a science: everything is not a clear-cut black or white; there are many grey areas. We are all one species; thus, for the most part whatever foods are good for one of us are good for all of us, and whatever diseases are harmful to one of us are harmful to all of us. However, we are all sufficiently individual that while some will suffer a disease during an epidemic, others will escape.

It is very unusual to find unanimity within the medical professions. Yet, for the most part, that is exactly what we appear to have had with fluoride for nearly half a century. It is particularly unusual in this case because, according to Dr Albert Schatz, '[M]any individuals with impeccable credentials in science, dentistry, and medicine have published incontrovertible evidence that fluoridation is harmful and does not reduce the incidence of dental caries.' [1] There are literally tens of thousands of papers that have found that fluoride in all its forms is harmful. Not just harmful to us, but to other mammals, reptiles, birds, fish, plant life, even the very atmosphere we live in (fluorides have contributed to formation of the ozone hole). The real question, therefore, is not: Why is it that some doctors and dentists oppose fluoridation? but: Why do so many still support it?

It is true that in any organisation there will always be some who do not see eye-to-eye with their colleagues or agree with the stance of their professional organisation. That is not the case with fluoride. Speak out against fluoride, and you are not merely someone with a different opinion: you are immediately an outcast, shunned and reviled by your peers.

This was illustrated in a letter from Donald Kennedy, later to become commissioner of the Food and Drug Administration, and Dr Paul Ehrlich of Stanford University. Written to the Editorial Board, *Consumer Reports*, US Consumers Union, 4 March 1969, it read:

> Many of the statements in the CR report on fluoridation are directly contradicted by readily available scientific research. Rather than weigh all new evidence as it appears, in a constant and critical reevaluation of the advisability of fluoridation, the promoting agencies –

most notably the US public health service and the American Dental Association – have chosen to ignore any research that does not support their claims. On occasion they have suppressed information with negative implications for fluoridation; and many reputable, responsible scientists and physicians have been reluctant to voice any doubts they might have about the measure, because of the charges of quackery and worse that have been leveled at those who have objected to fluoridation in the past.

The statement, 'fluorides in the amounts needed for decay prevention are unquestionably safe for people of all ages and for the chronically ill', is sheer fabrication . . . The statement, (fluoride) 'is toxic only in high concentrations that have no relevance to any conceivable use in a community's water', likewise shows a total disregard for readily available evidence. The amount of fluoride added to water averages one part per million (1 ppm), a concentration designed to provide each person with one milligram (1 mg) of fluoride per day – based on the shaky assumption that each person drinks a quart of water a day. The FDA has established 2 mg per day as the maximum safe dose; at levels of ingestion higher than that, there is a chance of cumulative harmful effects, after many years, at least in more sensitive individuals. Thus the daily dose of 1 mg doesn't allow much room for safety . . . In addition, however, to this slim safety factor, it has been demonstrated that drinking water is not the only source of fluoride in our daily intake.

Blow the whistle – and be sacked

Scientists around the world were and are appalled at the notion of adding a known cumulative, protoplasmic poison to drinking water. Damage to humans, animals, plants and aquatic life is well documented in the literature even at levels *less* than the 'optimal' 1 part per million. Many scientists insist that fluoridation is scientifically, medically and ethically unsound. But those who voice such opinions are intimidated, denigrated and vilified by the fluoride promoters; they are refused publication in journals; and they are sacked from their jobs. Opposing fluoridation is a very dangerous thing to do.

A dentist defects

The late Dr John Colquhoun was chief dental officer of the Department of Health for Auckland, president of the New Zealand Fluoridation Society and a fervent supporter of fluoride and fluoridation. However, he discovered a number of worrying signs that led him to question the advisability of fluoridation. As a result of what he discovered, he came out against fluoridation. He explained his reasons in a public lecture given in Fife, Scotland, on 4 September 1996.[2]

In Auckland, Colquhoun had noticed a dramatic decline in decay rates that was not confined to the fluoridated areas. In both the fluoridated and unfluoridated parts of the city, the declines were similar. It was suggested to him that this was due to the use of fluoride toothpaste by children living in the unfluoridated part of the city. But he knew that in the unfluoridated part, very few children used fluoride toothpaste, most had not received fluoride applications to their teeth, and hardly any had been given fluoride tablets.

When he received the figures for Auckland, Colquhoun said: 'To my horror, they showed that fewer fillings had been required in the unfluoridated part of Auckland than in the fluoridated part.' So he asked for the national figures for tooth decay rates of all 5-year-olds in New Zealand, obtained from dental clinics throughout the country for the period 1930–90, together with data on water fluoridation and fluoride toothpaste use.

In Figure 1, you can see what Dr Colquhoun saw after he had analysed the figures: there had been a decline in decay rates over the whole period – *beginning well before fluorides started to be used.*

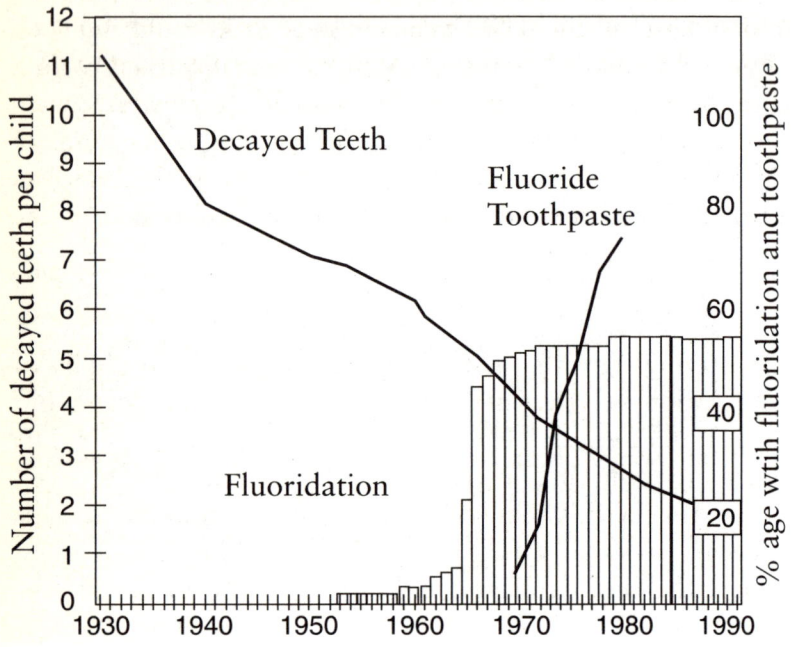

Source: Colquhoun J. *Perspect Biol Med* 1997; 41: 29–44.

Figure 1. Decay rates in 5-year-olds, flouridation and flouride toothpaste.

When Colquhoun received these figures, they came with a warning that they were not to be made public. Colquhoun realised why: 'They showed that in most Health Districts the percentage of children who were free of tooth decay was greater in the unfluoridated parts of the district.'

It was a great and courageous step on Dr Colquhoun's

part when he came out against fluoridation. He was 'retired' from his post in 1990.

Dr William Marcus

Dr William Marcus, PhD, was senior science advisor and chief toxicologist at the US Environmental Protection Agency's Office of Drinking Water. In 1990, he was disturbed to find data from a study on rats by Battelle Northwest which showed an increased level of bone cancer and other kinds of cancer in the animals. In a radio interview with American journalist and broadcaster Gary Null, Dr Marcus said:[3]

> When I got a hold of the contractor report and reviewed it very carefully . . . it was reporting cancers in the animals, osteosarcomas, which bothered me a lot because I've been trying to produce osteosarcomas in animals for almost twenty years and the only luck I ever had was with an experiment in dogs and monkeys, and the osteosarcomas took nearly the lifetime of the animals, and we were using radium which specifically produces that in bones, and here we have a compound commonly available (fluoride) that did it in rats in two years or less.
>
> Secondarily, in that same study, there were cancers of the liver that are very rare according to the board-certified veterinary pathologist at the contractor, Battelle, and those really were very upsetting because they were hepatocholangiocarcinoma, a very, very rare liver cancer . . . then there were several other kinds of cancers found in the jaw and other places . . . It showed that the levels of the fluoride that caused the cancers in the animals were actually lower than those levels seen in people who are ingesting lower amounts but for longer periods of time and that was very, very worrisome. It meant that the general population could be exposed to

fluoride known to cause cancer in animals and have levels near [those that caused] the cancer being produced in the bones.

In the USA, the law does not allow anything that has been shown to cause cancer in animals to be put in foods or drinks.

Dr Marcus went to the seminar at Research Triangle Park where representatives of the National Toxicology Program were presenting their review of the study. He attended with several colleagues, one of whom was a board-certified veterinary pathologist who had originally reported hepato-cholangiocarcinoma as a separate entity in rats and mice. Marcus asked him if he would look at the slides to check that the diagnosis was correct. It was. But at the meeting, Dr Marcus found that every one of the cancers that was reported by the contractor had been downgraded by the NTP. He said:

> Now I've been in the toxicology business looking at studies of this nature for nearly twenty-five years and I've never seen that, never ever seen where every single endpoint that was a cancer endpoint had been downgraded . . . I found that very suspicious . . . and found out that the scientists at the NTP down at Research Triangle Park had been coerced to change their findings.

Something was very wrong. Dr Marcus wrote a memo calling for a review of the cover-up of the National Toxicology Program study that shows fluoride is a 'probable human carcinogen'. He was promptly fired from his job at the EPA.

Later, an investigation by the Senate Environment and Public Works Committee corroborated his charges and produced evidence that government scientists had been pressured to portray fluoride more positively.

Dr Marcus endured a two-year lawsuit, which he won with punitive damages. He was then reinstated in his EPA job. Despite this, the classifications have never been reviewed.

Dr Phyllis J. Mullenix

Three days after she joyfully announced to the Forsyth Dental Institute that her neurotoxicity study (see Chapter 5) had been accepted for publication by the *Journal of Neurotoxicology and Teratology*, Dr Phyllis Mullenix was fired and all grants and funding for all her research projects stopped. The reason given by Forsyth for her dismissal was that her work was not 'dentally related'! The institute's director stated, according to Mullenix, that 'they didn't consider the safety or the toxicity of fluoride as being their kind of science'.[4] In which case, why was Dr Mullenix assigned the study of fluoride toxicity in the first place?

Both Forsyth and the National Institutes of Health wanted to know in which journal her research was to be published, but she refused to disclose that information because she knew that they would attempt to stop its publication.

Soon after her dismissal, Dr Mullenix said, the Forsyth Institute received a quarter-million dollar grant from the Colgate toothpaste company. Coincidence or reward? Mullenix's equipment and computers, designed specifically for the studies, were mysteriously damaged and destroyed by water leakage before she could remove them from Forsyth. Coincidence?

Dr Mullenix was then given an unfunded research position at Children's Hospital in Boston, but with no equipment and no money. Mullenix said, 'The people at Children's Hospital, for heaven's sake, came right out and said they were scared because they knew how important the fluoride issue was.'

Like Dr Marcus, Mullenix sued and won substantial punitive damages from her employers, but the career of this brilliant scientist was ruined because she found that fluoride was toxic.

Dr Allan S. Gray

Canadian dentist, Dr Allan S. Gray, found that the teeth of children in unfluoridated parts of British Columbia were in much better condition than those of children in the fluoridated areas.[5] For publishing that research, the top public health dentist in British Columbia was demoted and sent to Ottawa, where he was put in a basement office and ordered never to speak to anybody about the matter again. If he did, he was told, he would lose his standing in the public health department of Canada and very likely all of his retirement benefits.

Conclusion

These are just four highly qualified and highly principled scientists who have had the courage to stand against the blinkered, uncaring might of the fluoride establishment. They are not alone, as more and more are changing sides.

The BFS talks glibly of individuals who are 'out of step' with their professions. But there are hundreds of dentists and scientists in other specialisations who have come out against fluoride. One has only to look at the qualifications of some of those who oppose fluoridation to see that they are not uninformed laymen or even rank-and-file members of their professions. Many are eminent and respected scientists with a wide range of health and environmental specialities. Appendix A provides a random selection of highly qualified men and women who are prominent in their fields and who have spoken out against fluoridation. The appendix includes leading dentists, scientists in other disciplines and sixteen Nobel Prize winners. Such a listing makes absurd the claims of fluoride promoters that there is 'no scientific debate' over fluoridation and that the only people who are concerned about it are 'crackpots'.

References

1. Schatz A. Letter to Alderman Ray Jones, chairman, Operations and Environmental Committee, City of Calgary, 8 September 1997. http://www.cadvision. com/fluoride/calgary1.htm.

2. Colquhoun J. Why I changed my mind about water fluoridation. *Perspect Biol Med* 1997; 41: 1–16.

3. Marcus W. Radio interview with Gary Null, Program #310. Broadcast 10 March 1995. Access at http://www.sonic.net/~kryptox/medicine/cancer/ifin19.txt.

4. The dark odyssey of Dr Phyllis Mullenix. World Internet News Distributary Source. http://thewinds.org/archive/medical/fluoride01-98.html. Accessed 15 September 2000.

5. Gray AS. Time for a new baseline. *J Can Dent Assoc* 1987; 53: 763–5.

20. The Poor and Fluoride Toxicity

Dental health is improving, so why do we need fluoridation?

BFS suggested answer

Over the past 25 years or so tooth decay rates have improved largely due to the widespread use of fluoride toothpastes and greater awareness of sugar in the diet. However, the improvement has been greater among the more affluent and inequalities in dental health have widened – except where water supplies are fluoridated.

In non-fluoridated Glasgow for example, the single most common reason for children under the age of 10 needing a general anaesthetic is for tooth extraction. In the poorest parts of non-fluoridated Liverpool 1 in 3 young children have had teeth extracted before the age of 5. In Birmingham where the water has been fluoridated for 35 years such statistics are now unheard of.

Water fluoridation gives poor kids rich kids' teeth!

BFS suggested answer refuted

Poor, malnourished children, especially infants, are the most sensitive barometer of fluoride toxicity.
Dr Albert Schatz

In Britain and Ireland today, it is recognised that the poor are at greater risk of suffering from decayed teeth. The UK government's *Saving Lives: Our Healthier Nation* states:

> Poor people are ill more often and die sooner. To tackle
> these fundamental inequalities we must concentrate

attention and resources on the areas most affected by air pollution, poverty, low wages, unemployment, poor housing, crime and disorder, which can make people ill in both body and mind.

Dentists and health authorities are particularly anxious to target fluoride at areas of poverty, as it is among the poorer elements of society that the highest incidences of tooth decay are found. Unfortunately, evidence has shown that a good diet is essential if one is to mitigate the adverse effects of fluoride. People who have less than adequate diets – 'the poor' – are just the people who are most likely to be damaged by the very fluoride that is supposed to help them.

Children are the most susceptible to adverse health effects caused from the ingestion of chemically treated water. Children from families with good incomes suffer less from adverse health effects like dental fluorosis, while children from lower-income families are more likely to suffer adverse health effects.

Using instances of dental fluorosis as an indicator, poor children have 2.3 times as much fluorosis as children from higher-income families.[1] This ratio suggests that the toxic contaminants associated with fluorosilicic acid would also affect children's health to a similar degree. The reason for the disparity between economic brackets is nutrition: good nutrition provides enough minerals and vitamins to help the body counteract the adverse effects of fluoride.

Fluoride is of no benefit to the poor in England . . .

The BFS rightly makes the point that poor children tend to have a worse dental record than children in wealthier families. But that is the point they conveniently 'forget' when they compare decay rates in different towns. Any meaningful result requires comparisons between children with similar socio-economic profiles within fluoridated and unfluoridated areas.

It is no good comparing, for example, children from wealthy families living in a fluoridated area with children from poor families living in an unfluoridated area, and then claiming that the better teeth of the 'rich kids' are due to the fluoride. Yet, in comparing Glasgow and 'the poorest parts' of Liverpool with Birmingham, that is exactly what the BFS has done.

The amount of deprivation in an area, and thus the number of poorer children, is measured by the 'Jarman score', or UPA (underprivileged area) score. The higher the number, the more underprivileged it is. Let us try another comparison, this time between Liverpool, a northern seaport on the west coast of England, and Gateshead, a northern English seaport on the east coast:

- Based on the 1991 census, Gateshead's UPA score is 14.75, while Liverpool's is 34.69.[2] Thus, Liverpool's children are poorer, and one can expect that Liverpool children's teeth will have more decay.

- Gateshead's children drink artificially fluoridated water at the 'optimum' 1 ppm; Liverpool's water is not fluoridated. If fluoride helps teeth, as the BFS claims, this, again, should mean that Liverpool children's teeth should have more decay.

But this is not the case. The rates of dental caries in Liverpool and Gateshead, as measured by the British Dental Association, are identical: 5-year-olds have an average of 1.85 carious teeth in both cities.

. . . or in the USA

A survey of 39,000 children living in fluoridated, unfluoridated or partially fluoridated communities was conducted by the National Institute for Dental Research in 1986–87.[3] Although it cost US taxpayers $3.6 million, the data from this study were suppressed. Nevertheless, Dr John

Yiamouyiannis managed to pry the data out of the NIDR by using the Freedom of Information Act and, from the data, was able to show that there was a difference of less than half a tooth in DMFT values.

Is that enough to compensate for the stigma of stained teeth caused by dental fluorosis? Or the other more serious health effects? According to Dr Hardy Limeback, head of preventive dentistry at the University of Toronto, fluoridation of water 'has contributed to the birth of a multi-billion dollar industry of tooth bleaching and cosmetic dentistry. More money is being spent now on the treatment of dental fluorosis than what would be spent on dental decay if water fluoridation were halted.'[4]

Tooth decay is down – where nutrition is better

As was discussed in Chapter 1, the tooth decay rate has gone down in both fluoridated and unfluoridated communities all over Europe and America. It is not because of fluoride, and it is not because we are eating less sugar. The reason decay rates are declining is because we are eating more protein than our malnourished ancestors did, and we are focussing on dental hygiene as a social requirement. But high-protein foods – meat, fish, dairy products – are more expensive, and the poor are less able to afford them. So they survive largely on bread and potatoes, while their children, more than most, are comforted with sweetened dummies, sweets, colas: all the things that increase decay rates.

Studies from other parts of the world confirm this – and it has been known for a long time. In 1952, the *Journal of the American Dental Association* told its readers:

> The higher index of mottling in Italy may be explained on the basis of differences in nutritional status . . . The data from this and other investigations suggest that malnourished infants and children, especially if deficient

in calcium intake, may suffer from the effects of water containing fluorine while healthy children would remain unaffected.[5]

Maury Massler, professor of pedodontics at the University of Illinois College of Dentistry, warned that 'low levels of fluoride ingestion which are generally considered to be safe for the general population may not be safe for malnourished infants and children, because of disturbances in calcium metabolism'.[6]

Conclusion

What makes the efforts to fluoridate us all so pernicious is that they are being promoted in the name of protecting the poor. Yet it is well understood among fluoride researchers that it is precisely those who are malnourished, and consequently are likely to be the poor in our society, who are most vulnerable to, and most adversely affected by, fluoride's toxic effects.

Far from water fluoridation giving poor kids rich kids' teeth, as the BFS suggests, it seems that the opposite is true: fluoridation gives rich kids poor kids' teeth.

References

1. Taber, CW. *Taber's cyclopedic medical dictionary*, Philadelphia, F.A. Davis Co., 1994.
2. *1991 UPA scores by 1996 Health Authority boundaries*. Division of Primary Care and Population Health Sciences, Imperial College School of Medicine. http://www.med.ic.ac.uk/df/dfgm/upa/download.htm. Accessed 14 July 2000.
3. Yiamouyiannis JA. Water fluoridation and tooth decay: Results from the 1986–87 national survey of US schoolchildren. *Fluoride* 1990; 23: 55–67.

4. Limeback H. International Fluoride Information Network Bulletin No. 3. Available from ggvideo@northnet.org.
5. Relation of endemic dental fluorosis to malnutrition. *J Am Dent Assoc* 1952; 44: 182.
6. Should Natick Fluoridate? A report to the town and to the board of selectmen, Natick Fluoridation Study Committee. Natick, MA, 23 October 1997. http://www.cadvision.com/fluoride/natick.htm. Accessed 8 April 2000.

21. Sugar and Truth Decay

Why not just concentrate efforts on trying to make sure everyone eats less sugar and uses fluoride toothpaste?

BFS suggested answer
Although dental health has improved for many, but as a result inequalities in dental health have widened (*sic*). Changing people's behaviour is difficult and takes time. Meanwhile young children in our poorest communities continue to suffer high levels of avoidable disease.

Water fluoridation is the only measure we know of which will reduce tooth decay for everyone irrespective of behaviour.

BFS suggested answer refuted
Why is it that so many of the profession [dentists] who are preventively orientated are so frequently seen eating the biscuits richly embellished with jam, chocolate and sugar that are provided at virtually all meetings organized by dental societies, hospitals and members of the dental trade?
Elizabeth Elliott, executive manager, British Dental Health Foundation

It is generally accepted within medical circles that prevention is better than cure. Certainly we all seem to say that, even if we are not inclined to do much about it ourselves. Over the past couple of decades, our knowledge of how different foods affect our bodies has increased dramatically: we all know that if we didn't smoke, took more exercise, watched our diet, and so on, we would be healthier. Having said that, however, there are still many diseases that changing to a 'healthier' regime will not prevent.

Tooth decay is not one of them.

There is no need whatsoever for anyone to have decayed teeth. We know exactly what causes dental caries, and we know exactly how to prevent it: we've known it for decades. The problem is that dentists don't seem to want to tell us very forcefully. True, there is advice dished out in dentists' waiting rooms and by health authorities, generally built around three main pillars: brush your teeth regularly (with a fluoridated toothpaste, naturally); visit your dentist regularly; and don't eat sweets between meals. But it isn't very successful: people are still queueing up to get their teeth filled, capped, bridged or removed.

Half a century ago, toothpaste ingredients were all the rage: ingredients that purported to kill bacteria, or neutralise the acids made by the bacteria, or make your breath smell sweeter, but they never quite worked. Then came the magic ingredient: fluoride. All the chlorophyll, GL99, and abrasives, which had been the mainstay of toothpastes' supposed effectiveness, disappeared in favour of this new ingredient which promised 'fewer fillings'. Despite this dramatic change of emphasis, little else changed. The claims for this new wonder ingredient, just like those that went before, were still aimed at 'cure' rather than 'prevention'. And the basis of all the advice given has little real basis in fact.

Extravagant claims are made for fluoride, but dental advice is still based around the same three pillars – and it seems there is little evidence that these pillars have sound foundations. Before we look at these in detail, it would be as well to understand the process of decay.

Tooth decay

The smell of a baby's breath while it is breast feeding and before its teeth start to erupt is sweet and curiously attractive. But get to the teething stage, and all that begins to change.

The reason for this change is in the design of our mouths. Warm and moist, they are the ideal breeding ground for bacteria and minute yeasts. Nature has determined that under normal circumstances, if we eat a natural diet, the dominant bacteria are benign and, by crowding out more dangerous bacteria, protect our mouths. But when we eat foods that we are not designed to eat, we create a situation in which a class of bacteria that 'glue' themselves to our teeth and gums can thrive. It is these bacteria – principally *Streptococcus mutans* – that cause tooth decay. The 'glue', made from sugars and starches (carbohydrates) that we eat, is also their food supply. The combination of bacteria and glue is called 'plaque'.

In the middle ages and before, tooth decay was rare.[1] Nobody brushed their teeth in those days, levels of plaque were high, yet rates of decay were small. It was only among the rich that decay occurred earlier in life, as they could afford to buy prohibitively costly sugar.[2]

We have known since the Middle Ages that sugar is the cause of blackened, rotting teeth. Paul Hentzner, describing Elizabeth I, says she had 'a hooked nose, narrow lips and black teeth, a defect the English seem prone to from their too great use of sugar'. And Shakespeare in *Romeo and Juliet* writes: 'Because their breaths with sweetmeats tainted are'.

The three pillars of dental wisdom

The three pillars of dental advice should be looked at in more detail and revised:

- **Brush your teeth after meals.** We know that when teeth are exposed to a sugar solution, the acidity at the tooth rises to a dangerous level within one minute and stays at that strength for another twenty minutes.[3] So brushing teeth immediately after a meal seems like good advice. But how many people get up from the table immediately and brush their teeth – I mean immediately: within seconds? Professor G.N. Jenkins, in his standard work, *The Physiology of the Mouth*, published in 1956, says that it makes much more sense to brush teeth *before* eating a meal. Plaque bacteria feed on and ferment dietary sugars and starches. These bacteria start the process of acid formation immediately you start eating these foodstuffs. It is better to remove the bacteria before eating. That way there aren't any bacteria on the teeth to start the dental decay process during a meal.

- **Visit your dentist every six months.** According to dentists Richard and Elizabeth Cook, nobody knows how this one began. Certainly a study published in 1977 could find no scientific basis for the recommendation.[4] An American dentist, Jack Anderson,[5] managed to trace it back to the *Amos and Andy Show*, which was sponsored by the Ipana Toothpaste Company in the 1930s. Ipana's slogan was 'Brush with Ipana twice a day and visit your dentist twice a year.' But children who visit their dentists twice a year have no better teeth than people who go at greater intervals.[6] A Swedish study showed that people who visited their dentists more often merely ended up with more fillings.[7]

- **Don't eat sweets between meals.** This is very good advice with plenty of evidence to support it. If teeth are continually bathed in a solution of sugar, then the bacteria in plaque will produce acid continually. So don't eat sweets between meals. Don't drink pop and colas either. Or fruit juices, or bags of crisps, or biscuits, or bread. But how often and how loudly do we hear it? You will see adverts on TV for fluoridated toothpaste, but how many have you seen warning of the dangers of eating between meals? The truth is that dentists are trained to repair teeth. They are not trained to prevent cavities. So they promote fluoride instead. This, we are assured, will prevent dental decay. Use fluoride toothpastes and drink fluoridated water, and we can eat all the sweets we like with impunity.

Dentists make more money in fluoridated areas

Dentists make much more money in fluoridated areas. Fluorosis causes disfigurement: cosmetic dentistry is far more lucrative than cavity repair. Fluoride also causes a delay in the normal shedding of the baby teeth and their replacement by permanent teeth. This delay increases the number of children with malpositioned teeth, so today more braces are fitted. Braces are also far more lucrative than fillings.

Conclusion

As fluoridation is the easy option and dentists make more money in fluoridated areas, there is little incentive for dentists to instil healthier eating practices in their patients.

References

1. Moore WJ, Corbett ME. The distribution of dental caries in ancient British populations. *Caries Res* 1971; 5: 151–68; *Caries Res* 1973; 7: 139–53; *Caries Res* 1975; 9: 163–75.
2. Rushton MA. The teeth of Anne Mowbray. *Br Dent J* 1965; 119: 355–9.
3. Stephan RM. *J Am Dent Assoc* 1944; 27: 718.
4. Sheiham A. *Lancet* 1977; ii (27 Aug): 442.
5. Quoted in Cook R, Cook E. *Sugar off! A practical guide to sugar-free living.* London: Pan Books, 1983.
6. *Children's dental health in England and Wales.* London: HMSO, 1975.
7. Axelsson P, Lindhe J. *J Clin Perio.* 1978; 5:133–51.

22. Money Down the Drain

Who pays for fluoridation?

BFS suggested answer
The total cost of fluoridation is borne by the NHS, not the water company nor the consumer.

Water fluoridation is a highly cost-effective public health measure. In a recent study of strategies for reducing tooth decay, the University of York Health Economics Consortium concluded that 'the most cost-effective policy is fluoridation of water supplies'.

BFS suggested answer refuted
The figure given for cost effectiveness is calculated from the per capita expenditure for fluoridation chemicals, the average cost of a filling and a reduction in caries of 40%. Most of which collapses like a deck of cards when it is recognized that the reduction of caries is a 'statistical illusion'.
Richard G. Foulkes, MD

The BFS's suggested answer is disingenuous: You, the consumer, pay for fluoridation through your taxes. You pay for the fluoride that is put in the water, you pay for the equipment needed to meter it into the water, and you also pay for the British Fluoridation Society's propaganda machine, as it is funded by the Department of Health. The British Fluoridation Society received £117,000 from a hard-pressed NHS in 1997. In Ireland, too, water fluoridation is paid for by the taxpayer.

A waste of public resources

In 1974 the World Health Organization based its recommendations on fluoridation on an expectation that a fluoride-based preventative programme could result in a more than thirtyfold saving of money on dental care.[1] But far from saving money, fluoridation has been shown to be, in effect, a case of throwing money down the drain.

It is recognised by both sides of the argument, that the only people to benefit from water fluoridation are children up to the age of about twelve. But it is estimated that less than one-tenth of 1 per cent of all tap water is drunk by children of this age group. The rest is used by industry, for washing people, dishes, clothes and cars, for watering gardens, or is drunk by adults. Thus, for every £100 spent on water fluoridation, less than 10p reaches its target.

Added to this waste are the extra dental costs necessitated by the more complicated and expensive dental work that fluoride-damaged teeth require. Dentists may deny this, but it is easy to demonstrate the truth, merely by analysing regional trends in dental health expenditures in Britain (see Table 1). Doing so shows clearly that not only are there more dentists in fluoridated areas, but the amount spent per head of population is greater.

The most critical way to assess the effectiveness of fluoridation is to examine how much money is spent within regional Health Authority boundaries. For the purpose of this exercise, three UK regions, which have both fluoridated and unfluoridated communities within their areas, have been chosen for close examination of dental health costs. The picture that emerges from artificially fluoridated districts is that more fluoridation results in higher expenditure by the patient and, as most dentists today operate privately outside the NHS, more profit for the dentists.

District	Fluoride level (% affected, level)	Expenditure (GB£)			Dentists per 100,000
		Per child	Per adult	Combined	
East Anglia					
Suffolk	100 Nat., 0.1–0.95 ppm	12.10	22.37	20.02	32.8
NW Anglia	Not fluoridated	9.21	16.08	14.51	25.1
Northern England					
Newcastle & N. Tyneside	80% Art., Opt.	11.26	23.27	20.62	37.8
Gateshead & S. Tyneside	57% Art. + 24% Nat.	8.56	22.88	19.64	36.4
Sunderland	Not fluoridated	9.87	20.44	17.89	30.2
West Midlands					
Birmingham	100% Art., Opt.	12.10	24.21	21.08	32.8
Wolverhampton	32% Art., Opt.	7.57	21.53	18.11	29.0
Western England (affluent)					
Worcestershire	33–71% Art., Opt.	16.14	19.65	18.86	32.5
Shropshire	Not fluoridated	8.36	15.67	13.98	29.9

Note: Art., artificial; Nat., natural; Opt., optimal. 'Fluoride level' shows the percentage of the population affected and the level of fluoride received; 'Opt.' means the fluoride concentration in water was greater than 0.7 ppm. 'Expenditure' is the sum of all receipts received for 1997 divided by the size of the population, thus giving the average cost of dentistry per person. 'Dentists' are those who were practising at the end of 1996; the ratio is based on the size of the total population divided by the number of dentists. The population levels are estimated at mid-1996 levels.

Table 1. Comparison of dental expenditure in selected fluoridated and unfluoridated districts of the United Kingdom

- East Anglia has no artificial fluoridation schemes in place, but some water contains a noticeable amount of naturally occurring fluoride. It is important to consider the impact of *natural* fluoride on a population because of the claim that natural fluoride is better than artificial fluoride. Observations in this region do not support that claim. Unfluoridated north-west Anglia has 23.5 per cent fewer dentists per head, and dental costs are down by almost 30 per cent compared with naturally fluoridated Suffolk.

- The northern region is home to two flagships of fluoridation: Newcastle and Gateshead. Both fluoridated since 1968, this allows us to compare adult expenditure. Both have the most dentists and the highest expenditure per head of population anywhere in the region. The only other major industrial town is Sunderland, which is also the only genuinely unfluoridated part of the region. Sunderland wins on all counts: dentistry is less expensive, and there are fewer dentists per head. Why is it that Newcastle and Gateshead have so many extra dentists if, as they claim, fluoridation reduces the need for them?

- West Midlands: Districts in this region are the 'shining' examples of the benefits of fluoridation, with Birmingham as the jewel in the crown. But expenditure in Birmingham is significantly higher than in less fluoridated Wolverhampton (all areas have some fluoridation). Wolverhampton is now 100 per cent fluoridated. It will be interesting to see how expenditure levels change and how many more dentists are drafted into the city to improve dental health.

- The western region: This part of England is significantly richer than the other regions examined. We can expect that teeth will be better and that less money will have to be spent on dental care. This proves to be the case. Again, there is a significant increase in the cost of dental care in the fluoridated part of the region.

Fluoridation is not cost-effective

According to Dr Hardy Limeback, more money is spent on treatment of dental fluorosis than on dental decay.'
It is easy to see why.

- It is accepted, even by the BFS, that a large proportion of children living in fluoridated areas suffer from dental fluorosis. Whether this is merely a cosmetic condition or a symptom of something more serious was discussed in Chapter 15, but either way, it is not aesthetically pleasing. Children with dental fluorosis need veneers to cover and hide their stained teeth – and a veneer is vastly more expensive than having a cavity filled.

- Fluoridation doesn't stop cavities. Children in fluoridated areas still suffer dental decay. When these cavities need to be repaired, it generally costs more because the fluoride makes teeth brittle – and they have a tendency to shatter.

Put your money where your mouth is

Almost all the fluoride that the taxpayer purchases to put in tap water doesn't reach its target; it merely pollutes the environment. If we choose to ignore the risks of fluoride and set as our goal the adequate provision of fluoride for children's teeth, the most sensible way to do it would be to use toothpaste and the numerous fluoride-containing dental products. For families who can't afford toothpaste, it would be more cost-effective for governments to provide these families with fluoride tablets or toothpaste. A policy of disseminating fluoride to the needy in this way would not only save money, it would have the added ethical advantage that much less toxic waste would enter the environment – and people who didn't want fluoridated water would not be forced to drink it.

References

1. Davies GN. *Cost and benefit of fluoride in the prevention of dental caries.* Offset Publication, No 9. WHO, 1974.

23. The History of Water Fluoridation, Part One

> ## Is it true that fluoridation is simply a way for industries to get rid of their toxic waste?
>
> **BFS suggested answer**
> It is not true. Water fluoridation is a proven SAFE AND EFFECTIVE PUBLIC HEALTH MEASURE to reduce tooth decay.
>
> **BFS suggested answer refuted**
> *Of course there were also those gigantic financial benefits for the industries who could at least sell a poisonous waste product for stupendous amounts of money.*
> Dr Hans Moolenburgh

Fluorine

Fluorine (F), a member of the halogen group of elements, is a pale yellow gas. It is never found on its own in nature but always bound to other elements in compounds called fluorides. The three most common sources of fluoride are: calcium fluoride, or fluorspar, a beautiful cubic glasslike crystal, in a variety of colours, found in England, Germany, Iceland, Mexico and Newfoundland (a deep blue variety from which vases and other ornaments are made, found in Derbyshire, England, is called Blue John); cryolite, or aluminium fluoride, found in Colorado, USA, Greenland, Russia and Spain; and fluorapatite, a complex calcium phosphate compound, found in Florida, Tennessee, and South Carolina, USA, South Africa and the West Indies.[1] The form of fluoride that is found naturally in fresh water is calcium fluoride.

Industry's toxic problem

During the nineteenth century, iron and copper factories' chimneys belched fluorides into the air, poisoning animals, plants and people.[2] The effects were devastating, particularly to agriculture. The first damages were paid in 1855 by iron smelters in Freiburg, Germany. In 1893 damages for injuries from fluoride contamination cost over DM700,000, and by 1900, the very existence of the smelting industry, both in Germany and Great Britain, was threatened.[3] By the 1920s, rapid industrial growth meant unimaginable pollution in the USA, Britain and other industrial countries. Medical writer Joel Griffiths explains that 'it was abundantly clear to both industry and government that spectacular US industrial expansion – and the economic and military power and vast profits it promised – would necessitate releasing millions of tons of waste fluoride into the environment'.[4] It didn't affect just commerce: the armed forces could not function without the tools of war – tools that simply could not be made if the toxic fluoride waste generated could not be disposed of.

The Mellon connection

The American Mellon family founded the Aluminum Company of America (ALCOA), one of the biggest fluoride polluters. When smelting and reducing aluminium, bauxite (aluminium ore) is dissolved in molten cryolite. This releases hydrogen fluoride gas and other volatile compounds into the atmosphere, while sodium fluoride remains in the bath.[5] Hydrogen fluoride, or hydrofluoric acid (HF), is so powerful an acid that it even etches glass. Dr Jag Cook, a member of Britain's National Chemical Emergency Group, which is responsible for dealing with disasters involving toxic chemicals, says, 'Hydrogen fluoride is about the only chemical that really frightens me.'[6] None of these substances could be dumped with impunity into the environment. Their disposal was expensive. It became imperative that industry find a way to eliminate, or at least reduce, these costs.

When the connection between fluorosis and fluoride was first made, American dentists had called for the removal of fluoride from water supplies. But in 1928, Dr Frederick S. McKay observed that teeth affected by fluorosis seemed less susceptible to dental caries.[7] Surveys funded by the US public health service, under the direction of the then US Treasury Secretary, Andrew W. Mellon, ALCOA's founder, appeared to reveal fewer cavities among children living in naturally fluoridated communities.

Public health service dental surgeon and epidemiologist Henry Trendley Dean led one of the three research teams. He became such a fervent researcher at that time that he is now known as 'the father of fluoridation'. In a major study of twenty-one cities in Colorado, Illinois, Indiana and Ohio, Dean reported that communities which had 0.9–1.4 ppm fluoride in their drinking water had only one-third as much dental decay as cities with less than 0.4 ppm fluoride,[8] and suggested 'the possibility of partially controlling dental caries through the domestic water supply'.[9]

In 1938, Dr Gerald Cox, a biochemist at the University of Pittsburgh's Dental School, and colleagues at the Mellon Institute, founded in 1913 to advance science and industry, claimed that fluoride, in small quantities, was not harmful and suggested that '[t]he present trend toward complete removal of fluoride from water may need some reversal'.[10] Dean had been working with water naturally fluoridated with calcium fluoride, but Cox fluoridated some laboratory rats with sodium fluoride (ALCOA's waste), concluded that fluoride reduced cavities, and said: 'The case should be regarded as proved.' A proposal was aired to add sodium fluoride to the entire nation's drinking water. While the dose to each individual would be low, 'fluoridation' on a national scale would require hundreds of thousands of tons of fluoride annually.

Not surprisingly, industry and the US government strongly supported the Mellon Institute's recommendation. In 1939, the first public proposal that the US should fluoridate its water supplies was made – not by a doctor, or dentist, but by a scientist working for a company threatened with huge claims for fluoride damage.

In 1950 ALCOA advertised: 'ALCOA sodium fluoride is particularly suitable for the fluoridation of water supplies . . . If your community is fluoridating its water supply – or is considering doing so – let us show you how ALCOA sodium fluoride can do the job for you.'[11]

But the 'waste' definition was a problem. In 1955 ALCOA denied that sodium fluoride was a waste product of aluminium manufacture. 'We make no direct sales of sodium fluoride, all of our production being handled through chemical distributors,' they said, as if the handling by a wholesaler somehow changed the origin of the product.[12] Doctors and dentists were persuaded to endorse the new health measure. Having once declared that fluoride was perfectly safe and had a wide margin of safety, it would be difficult for them to do a U-turn later without losing face. Now anyone who opposed this new 'health-enhancing' initiative for the benefit of small children could be derided as a quack. Reputable scientists who expressed their concern were listed with convicted felons and the Ku Klux Klan, and open scientific debate was stifled. It was one of the greatest public relations coups of all time.

The first experiment at Grand Rapids

In 1945 Grand Rapids, Michigan, became the first US city to be fluoridated. This was to be the intervention group in a ten-year study, with unfluoridated Muskegon as the control group. The hypothesis to be tested was that 'a concentration of about 1 part per million of fluoride in the drinking water, mechanically added, inhibits the development of dental caries in the user'.

Dr Philip Sutton of the Dental School of the University of Melbourne did a meticulously detailed review of this study, showing the errors and omissions that invalidated its results.[13] For example:

- Water supplies to both populations were not similar.

- The Grand Rapids groups varied in number from 1,806 children to 3 children; in Muskegon, fewer than 20 children were examined in twelve of the categories, and one 'group' consisted of just one child.

- Different methods of sampling were used in the two cities.

- The trial was of insufficient duration to measure any change in permanent teeth.

An American Dental Association press release telling of a reduction in tooth decay in Grand Rapids as a result of fluoridation was deceptive advertising – there had also been a similar decline in Muskegon *without* fluoride.[14]

The Grand Rapids experiment was supposed to last for ten years to allow sufficient time for health benefits or hazards to be evaluated. In 1946, however, just one year into the experiment, six more US cities adopted fluoridation without waiting for the results. In 1947, eighty-seven more communities were fluoridated. Such haste may seem surprising until we learn that in 1947 an ALCOA lawyer was appointed to head the public health service. He launched a campaign to change fluoride's image. 'Almost overnight . . . the popular image of fluoride – which at the time was being widely sold as rat and bug poison – became that of a beneficial provider of gleaming smiles, absolutely safe, and good for children, bestowed by a benevolent paternal government. Its opponents were permanently engraved on the public mind as crackpots and right-wing loonies,' writes Griffiths.

Other trials

There were several other trials in the USA and Canada. There are marked deficiencies and omissions in the compilation and reporting of data in all.

Newburgh, to be fluoridated with sodium fluoride, and unfluoridated Kingston are two cities about thirty miles apart in New York State. They were said to be comparable in all ways, including water supplies. But an analysis of the two cities' water supplies, carried out by the US Geological Survey, showed them to be of quite different composition: Newburgh's water contained nearly six times as much calcium and four times as much magnesium as Kingston's water. Calcium and magnesium are known to mitigate the effects of fluoride. Different methods of data collection and result presentation were used. There were changes in examiners and statisticians. There was uncertainty about population shifts in both cities.

In 1956 the study's final report found in favour of fluoride.

In May 1989, Dr J.V. Kumar and colleagues at the New York State Department of Health published a follow-up study that revealed that dental decay declined in both Newburgh and Kingston.[15] The difference in terms of DMFT for 7- to 14-year-old children was less than one tooth. And by 1995, the average number of DMFTs in Kingston, which was still unfluoridated, was slightly better than in fluoridated Newburgh – and Kingston had only half the level of dental fluorosis.[16]

Fluoridation marches on

The McCarthy era after World War II saw witch-hunts to uncover 'communists' within American society. Those who questioned the benefits of fluoride were now branded not just as quacks, but as left-wing subversives.

By 1950, fluoridation's image was a sterling one, and there was not much science could do to stop it. The public health service, established to protect the health of US citizens, was caught in a trap of its own making: having publicly promoted fluoride and funded it with taxpayers' money, the health authorities risked losing face if fluoridation were found to be unsafe and ineffective and laws were repealed, since scientists, politicians, dentists and physicians unanimously supported fluoride.[17] Consequently, proper studies concerning the effects of fluoride were not undertaken. Dr George Waldbott summed up the situation when he said that from the beginning, the controversy over fluoridating water supplies was 'a political, not a scientific health issue'.[18]

Disinformation and 'Newspeak'

Leading those who were pushing for universal fluoridation at that time was a Wisconsin dentist, J.J. Frisch. Frisch, with the support of Frank Bull, director of dental education for the Wisconsin State Board of Health, organised political campaigns to persuade local government officials to approve fluoridation. They successfully lobbied the American Dental Association and the United States public health service and, with the support of these bodies, removed any doubts that the public might have had about this new 'wonder drug'. In 1950, long before any studies into the safety or efficacy of fluoridating drinking water had been carried out, fluoridation of drinking water was deemed beneficial and safe.

At a conference in Washington, DC, in 1951, Dr Bull gave a keynote speech about how to get fluoridation accepted and discredit any opponents. Bull talked about the terminology to be used by pro-fluoridationists. They were to overcome the problem of dental fluorosis by calling it 'eggshell teeth', 'the most beautiful looking teeth that anyone ever had'. 'Artificial fluoridation' was to become 'controlled fluoridation', and they should never use the word 'experiment'. 'In Wisconsin', Bull said, 'we set up "demonstrations". They weren't experiments.' On adverse effects of fluoride, Bull said:

> Now in regard to toxicity – I noticed that Dr Bain used the term 'adding sodium fluoride'. We never do that. Sodium fluoride is rat poison. You add fluorides. Never mind that sodium fluoride business . . . If it is a fact that some individuals are against fluoridation, you have just got to knock their objections down. The question of toxicity is on the same order. Lay off it altogether. Just pass it over. 'We know there is absolutely no effect other than reducing tooth decay,' you say and go on.[19]

Bull knew that fluoride caused cancer – and covered it up. Later he said: 'With regard to cancer, when this thing came out we never mentioned it in Wisconsin.' Bull's speech revealed the key emphasis of fluoride promotion – they were not to use the scientific evidence, only propaganda.

Not long after this conference, a number of symposia were held. A notable one, set up by the American Association for the Advancement of Science in 1952, had in its preface: 'The eminent qualifications of each of the chapter authors should be sufficient evidence as to the high caliber and unbiased authenticity of the content.'[20] All participants, however, were fervent supporters of fluoridation. No-one opposed to fluoride was allowed to take part.

The Commission on Chronic Illness endorsed the recommendations. It is significant that the chairman of this committee was the same man – K.F. Maxcy, professor of public health at Johns Hopkins University, Baltimore, Maryland.[21]

The National Academy of Sciences and the National Research Council

The US National Research Council committee that considered fluoride, also chaired by Professor Maxcy, had nine members. These included three other scientists with close connections with fluoride-promoting industries: H. Trendley Dean, who had supplied much of the data on which fluoridation was based – hardly an impartial observer; B.G. Bibby, director of the Eastman Dental Dispensary of Rochester, New York, who had done research for the Sugar Research Foundation, Inc.; and F.F. Heyroth, assistant director of the Kettering Laboratory, which was financed by ALCOA. Their 'evidence' that fluoridation was harmless was that three million people had been drinking naturally fluoridated water for generations![22]

The American Medical Association is duped

In 1943 F.J. McClure, a biochemist working for the National Institute of Dental Research, estimated that the typical American diet contained 0.3–0.5 mg fluoride. McClure acknowledged that excess fluoride could have adverse side effects when he wrote: 'The data suggest that these [4.0–5.0 mg fluoride daily] may be the limits of fluorine which may be ingested daily [by healthy adults] without an appreciable hazard of body storage of fluorine.'[23] Nevertheless, in 1951, McClure convinced the American Medical Association's Council on Pharmacy and Chemistry, as well as its Council on Foods and Nutrition, that adding fluoride to drinking water was not hazardous.[24]

A third of the AMA delegates did vote against fluoridation. But an 'endorsement in principle' was passed, and this was taken to mean that the AMA supported fluoridation without reservation. With AMA backing, there was no stopping fluoridation. All who opposed fluoridation were shouted down. A member of the US House of Delegates wrote to Dr Waldbott in 1957: 'To oppose fluoridation openly is political suicide' – a situation that, sadly, still obtains today.

WHO endorsement of fluoridation

In 1958 the WHO set up a committee to look at fluoridation. The deck was already stacked, as five of the committee's seven members had promoted fluoridation in their respective countries. Research documenting poisoning from fluoridated water was rejected. Yet WHO did not endorse fluoridation at that time.

Despite cautions from G. Penso of the Italian delegation, who warned about 'possible genetic damage to future generations', in 1969 a motion to 'examine the possibility of introducing fluoridation' where 'fluoride intake is below optimum levels' was carried at the end of business, when only 45 of the 1,000 delegates were present.[25] There was also a request to the director-general of the WHO to 'continue to encourage research into the etiology of dental caries, the fluoride content of diets, and into the effects of greatly excessive intake of fluoride from natural sources'.

In 1975, a report was presented to the 28th World Assembly.[26] The report is notable in that it is little more than propaganda for fluoridation. The fundamental question of what level, if any, of fluoride ingestion is optimal was ignored. Despite this, the WHO began a programme to promote fluoridation of water supplies.

Fluoride comes to Britain

In Britain, there were also studies that purported to demonstrate that fluoride in the water resulted in a reduced incidence of decay. Hartlepool,[27] a town whose drinking water contained a naturally occurring fluoride level of 2 ppm, was compared with York, which was not fluoridated. The lower incidence of dental caries in Hartlepool was ascribed to the fluoride in its water supply.

Throughout any country, it is not difficult to find a variety of levels of tooth decay in both fluoridated and unfluoridated areas. If one picks a fluoridated area with a low level of tooth decay and an unfluoridated area with a high level, disregarding any other differences between them, it is not difficult to 'prove' that fluoride prevents caries.

But there are several comparable districts, fluoridated and unfluoridated, where levels of carious teeth are the same. Gateshead and Liverpool are demographically quite similar, and both have 1.85 carious teeth per child. But Gateshead is 100 per cent fluoridated, whereas Liverpool is unfluoridated.

So when comparing towns like Hartlepool and York, one has to look more closely at other possible confounding factors. Doing this, we find that in the 1960s, when the study was conducted, the biggest employer in York was the sweets manufacturer Rowntree. Rowntree's employed a sizeable proportion of the city's population. Not only were its workers allowed to eat as much confectionery as they wished while they were at work, they were also allowed to collect all the bits left over at the end of the week to take home. Thus, it is likely that their friends and relatives also had a higher intake of sweets than most. It is just as likely, therefore, that the reason York had a higher dental decay rate than Hartlepool was simply its greater intake of caries-causing sweets.

The British learn from America

Britain had sent a team of four dentists to the USA during the early part of 1952 to look at their studies.[28] When they returned to the United Kingdom, all were fervent supporters of fluoridation.

Enoch Powell was the first British Minister of Health to recommend the fluoridation of public water supplies, saying: 'There are no authoritative criticisms of fluoridation.' But many British scientists were against its introduction in Britain:

- Dr Hugh Sinclair, fellow of Magdalen College, Oxford, was concerned in 1963 about the 'entirely new principle that the public should in general be forced to consume something believed by the government to be good for them'.[29]

- The British Medical Association's chief press officer in 1964 stated: 'The British Medical Association regard fluoridation as a preventive medical treatment.' But as Lord Douglas of Barloch pointed out: 'Doctors are not permitted by our laws to operate on patients or to force drugs on patients against their will. If our law does not permit this, why should it be considered right for a water supply authority to put drugs in the water supply, which admittedly are of no value if consumed by the adult population and which cannot be proved to be safe.'

People in the know didn't want fluoride, and most others were suspicious. Nevertheless, in the 1960s and 1970s, proponents managed to get water companies to fluoridate the water supplies to a total of about 9 per cent of English residents.

Scotland

Fluoride has never been accepted in Scotland, and English laws do not apply there. In a landmark legal case brought against the Strathclyde Regional Council in 1983, Lord Jauncey ruled that water fluoridation was medicinal and therefore unlawful.[30] While this judgement applied only to Scotland, it set a precedent for the rest of the United Kingdom. So in 1985, the Conservative government changed the law. However, since that change no new fluoridation project has been started. At a judicial review in the High Court over the refusal of Northumbrian Water Plc to fluoridate its water supply in 1998, Justice Collins ruled that Northumbrian Water 'is perfectly entitled to refuse to fluoridate'.[31] This is the present situation.

Ireland

All natural sources of water in Ireland are low in fluoride. This was a golden opportunity for the US public health service to 'improve' the situation by introducing artificial fluoridation to the Irish. Funded by the US public health service, the Irish fluoridation law was passed in 1960 with almost no public consultation. A legal challenge in 1963 failed in the High Court, and subsequently in the Supreme Court. The government legal team defending fluoridation was helped by US government agencies.[32]

Fluoridation started in 1964, and the Republic of Ireland is now probably the most fluoridated country on earth. Today, 75 per cent of public water in Ireland is fluoridated with hydrofluorosilicic acid imported from The Netherlands – a country in which water fluoridation is banned.

Fluoride is a US export flop

Since the inception of fluoridation in the USA, its advocates have attempted to get fluoride accepted throughout the world. Yet despite the apparently overwhelming enthusiasm for fluoridation in the USA, the rest of the world has not been so easy to fool, and acceptance of this 'health' measure outside the USA has been decidedly limited.

During the 1950s and 1960s, the United States public health service gave millions of American taxpayers' dollars to Western European countries, including the United Kingdom, Ireland, Australia, New Zealand and Canada, in a huge push to promote fluoridation. UK and Irish institutions received at least the following sums:[33]

	1958	1960	1963
Ireland	$19,078	$62,250	$78,730
UK	$232,035	$900,048	$2,751,215

Poster campaigns proliferated in hospitals, doctors' and dentists' surgeries, libraries, schools and work canteens. Yet despite this effort, most of continental Europe dismissed fluoride outright, and of those countries that tried it, almost all have given it up, and some have banned it outright (see Chapter 27).

Conclusion

A more truthful answer to this question would be: Yes. It is precisely because industry had a vexing and costly toxic-waste problem that fluoride began to be put in tap water. The fluoride compounds used to fluoridate drinking water do not include naturally occurring calcium fluoride. They are not 'simply the fluoride ion in water'; they constitute a complex cocktail of toxic substances that most countries have labelled as hazardous air pollutants.

References

1. Waldbott GL, in collaboration with Burgstahler AW, McKinney HL. *Fluoridation: The great dilemma*. Lawrence, KS: Coronado Press, 1978: 21–2.
2. Griffiths J. Fluoride: Commie plot or capitalist ploy. *Covert Action* 1992; 42: 27.
3. Ost H. The fight against injurious industrial gases. *Z Angew Chem* 1907; 20: 1689–93.
4. Griffiths J. Fluoride: Commie plot or capitalist ploy. *Covert Action* 1992; 42: 28.
5. Davenport SJ, Morris GG. *US Bureau of Mines Circular No. 7687*. US Department of the Interior, June 1954: 8.
6. Cook J. Quoted in Townson N, Campbell D. Deadly risks of lead-free petrol. *New Statesman*, 20 October 1988.
7. McKay FS. Relation of mottled enamel to caries. *J Am Dent Assoc* 1928; 15: 1429–37.
8. Dean HT. *Epidemiological studies in the United States*. In: Moulton FR, ed. *Dental caries and fluorine*. Washington, DC: American Association for the Advancement of Science, 1946.

9. Dean HT. Endemic fluorosis and its relation to dental caries. *Public Health Rep* 1938; 53: 1443–52.

10. Griffiths J. Fluoride: Commie plot or capitalist ploy. *Covert Action* 1992; 42: 28.

11. *J Am Water Works Assoc* 1950; 43 (6).

12. *J Am Dent Assoc* 1955; 51: 373.

13. Sutton PRN. *Fluoridation: Errors and omissions in experimental trials.* Melbourne University Press: Melbourne, 1959.

14. Maxcy KF, Appleton JLT, Bibby BG. *Report of the Ad Hoc Committee on Fluoridation of Water Supplies.* Publication No. 214, National Academy of Sciences/US National Research Council, 1952.

15. Kumar VK, Green EL, Wallace W, Carnahan T. Trends in dental fluorosis and dental caries prevalences in Newburgh and Kingston, New York. *Am J Public Health* 1989; 79: 565–9.

16. Kumar JK, Swango PA, Lininger LL et al. Changes in dental fluorosis and dental caries in Newburgh and Kingston, New York. *Am J Public Health* 1998; 88: 1866–70.

17. *Morning Call*, Allentown, Pennysylvania, 7 February 1990.

18. Waldbott GL, in collaboration with Burgstahler AW, McKinney HL. *Fluoridation: The great dilemma.* Lawrence, KS: Coronado Press, 1978: 255.

19. Proceedings of the Fourth Annual Conference of State Dental Directors with the Public Health Service and the Children's Bureau, Federal Security Building, Washington, DC, USA, 6–8 June 1951.

20. Shaw JH, ed. *Fluoridation as a public health measure.* Washington, DC: American Association for the Advancement of Science, 1954: iv–v.

21. Maxcy KF et al. *Report of the Ad Hoc Committee on Fluoridation of Water Supplies.* Publication No. 214,

National Academy of Sciences/US National Research Council, 1952.

22. Waldbott GL, in collaboration with Burgstahler AW, McKinney HL. *Fluoridation: The great dilemma.* Lawrence, KS: Coronado Press, 1978: 276.

23. McClure FJ, Mitchell HH, Hamilton TS, Kinser CA. Balances of fluorine ingested from various sources in food and water by five young men. Excretion of fluorine through the skin. *J Ind Hyg Toxicol* 1945; 27: 159–70.

24. American Medical Association Councils on Pharmacy and Chemistry and Foods and Nutrition: Fluoridation of water supplies. *J Am Med Assoc* 1951; 147: 1359.

25. WHO. Resolution of the World Health Assembly: Fluoridation and dental health. *WHO Chronicle* 1969; 23: 512.

26. Barmes DE, Infirri SJ. WHO activities in oral epidemiology: Global Oral Epidemiology Data Bank. *Community Dent Oral Epidemiol* 1977; 5(1): 22–9.

27. Murray J. Adult dental health in fluoride and non-fluoride areas. *Br Dent J* 1971; 131: 437–42.

28. Forrest JR, Longwell J, Stones HH, Thomsom AM. *The fluoridation of domestic water supplies in North America as a means of controlling dental caries.* London: HMSO, 1953.

29. *Oxford Times* (United Kingdom), 15 February 1963.

30. Lord Jauncey (1983): Opinion of Lord Jauncey in *Causa Mrs Catherine McColl (AP) v Strathclyde Regional Council,* The Court of Session, Edinburgh, 29 June 1983.

31. Judicial review sought by Newcastle Upon Tyne Health Authority, November 1998.

32. Waldbott GL. *A struggle with titans.* New York: Carlton Press, 1965.

33. Public Health Service, Grants and Fellowships. US Dept. of HEW, PHS, Publ 621 (1958); Publ 777, PT1 (1960); Publ 1075 PT1 (1963).

24. Arsenic and Old Lies

Is it true that the fluoride added to the water is not the same as that which occurs naturally?

BFS suggested answer
It is not true. Fluoride ions in solution in water are identical whether they occur naturally in the water or are added.

BFS suggested answer refuted
Hydrofluosilicic acid . . . is derived from toxic gases produced in the manufacture of phosphoric acid and phosphate fertilizers; it contains lead, mercury, arsenic, and high concentrations of radionucloides; it is also the chemical agent most used for water fluoridation in the United States.
George Glasser

The truth? The whole truth? – It's nothing like the truth

It's obvious from the BFS's answer that its members are not chemists. The element, fluorine, is the same, but when it comes with other elements, its effect on our bodies can be quite different. For example: the deadly nerve gas sarin, isopropyl-methyl-phosphoryl fluoride, is a 'fluoride'.

The fluoride compounds used to fluoridate drinking water are a complex cocktail of toxic substances that most countries have labelled 'hazardous air pollutants' (see Chapter 25). And their actions in the body differ considerably. Fluorine will form compounds with many different elements, but the bonds it forms are stronger with some than with others.

In 1935, C.H. Kick and colleagues fed different fluoride compounds to rats.[1] Measuring the amounts of fluorine ingested and excreted, they were able to calculate how much fluorine the rats absorbed and how much of that was retained in their bodies. The study's results, shown in Table 1, show the vast difference between the various compounds. The rats absorbed only 1.7 per cent (4.1 mg) of the fluorine from the naturally occurring calcium fluoride and retained none of it. This was not the case with the other compounds. With sodium fluoride, some 44.8 per cent (94.7 mg) of the fluorine was absorbed and almost a third retained, while 65 per cent (175.5 mg) of the fluorine in the fluorosilicate was absorbed, with again almost a third retained. The fluorine the rats retained was incorporated in bone and other tissue and thus accumulated in their bodies.

Fluorine supplement	Time fed (days)	Fluorine ingested (mg)	Fluorine in faeces (mg)	Fluorine in urine (mg)	Fluorine absorbed (mg)	Fluorine balance (mg)	Fluorine retained (%))
Sodium fluorosilicate (Na_2SiF_6)	22	269.9	94.4	90.2	175.5	85.3	31.6
Sodium fluoride (NaF)	18	211.2	116.5	25.8	94.7	68.9	32.6
Calcium fluoride (CaF_2)	11	229.6	225.5	4.2	4.1	−0.1	0

Source: Kick et al. *Fluorine in animal nutrition.* Ohio Agricultural Experiment Station, Bulletin 558, November 1935: 61.

Table 1. *Retention of fluorine in rats after ingestion of various fluoride compounds*

Kaj Roholm and George Waldbott also make a distinction between the relative toxicity of different fluoride compounds:

Comparison of toxicity of inorganic fluorides:[2]

Extremely toxic

Gaseous hydrogen fluoride   HF
Silicon tetrafluoride SiF_4

Solutions of hydrofluoric acid   HF
Hydrofluorosilicic acid H_2SiF_6

Very toxic

Easily soluble fluorides and fluorosilicates:
Sodium fluoride   NaF
Potassium fluoride   KF
Ammonium fluoride NH_4F
Sodium fluorosilicate Na_2SiF_6
Potassium fluorosilicate K_2SiF_6
Ammonium silicofluoride $(NF_4)_2SiF_6$

Moderately toxic

Almost insoluble fluoride compounds:
Cryolite Na_3AlF_6
Calcium fluoride CaF_2

When tests were done in the early part of the century to determine how much fluoride was 'safe' or 'optimal', they were conducted using the calcium fluoride that occurred naturally in water. But that is not the compound that is used either in water fluoridation or in toothpastes, gels and mouthwashes. As yet – and let's not forget that water has been artificially fluoridated for over half a century – no test has ever been carried out to determine what, if any, level of sodium fluoride, sodium fluorosilicate or hydrofluoric acid is the safe or optimal level.

So why not use calcium fluoride to fluoridate drinking water?

One reason that some 'fluorides' are more toxic than others lies in the strength of the bonds between the various atoms in the compounds. In the organic form – calcium fluoride (CaF_2) – the two fluorine atoms form a very strong bond with the calcium atom; a bond which is not easily broken. This makes the fluorine relatively inert and less likely to dissociate itself and form compounds with other minerals within the body. This is why it is less toxic.

But if this is so, why is calcium fluoride not used to fluoridate water? The cynic might answer that as this is not an industrial waste product looking for an outlet, but a natural chemical that would have to be mined, it is relatively more expensive. But there is another advantage to using the more toxic inorganic fluorides: unlike them, calcium fluoride is not very soluble in water.

Arsenic

Not only is the fluoride itself nearly as toxic as arsenic, but the results of tests also indicate that the most common contaminant detected in the fluoridation product is arsenic. Arsenic is a known carcinogen. There is no argument about it. Chronic health effects at low concentrations of arsenic include prostate, skin, bladder and lung cancers and a wide range of other conditions.

The product used to fluoridate water, derived as it is from phosphate fertiliser waste, is not pure. It is contaminated with arsenic and several other potentially dangerous elements. This fact prompted US Senator Bob Smith to call a senate hearing on 29 June 2000. The US EPA suggested a reduction in the maximum contaminant level (MCL) of arsenic from 50 parts per billion (ppb) to 5 ppb.

A 5 ppb arsenic standard would prevent about 50,000 cases of bladder cancer and approximately 12,500 bladder cancer deaths per year. But it would also result in the lowering of the maximum allowable level (MAL) of arsenic in the fluoridation product. The National Sanitation Foundation Inc showed that the average arsenic levels in the fluoridation agent were already well above the MAL.[3] At a cost of $445 million, a 5 ppb arsenic level would effectively kill off fluoridation.

Consequently, the EPA are considering a compromise 10 ppb standard in the MCL. This will allow more arsenic and prevent fewer cancers – about 32,500 cases of bladder cancer and 7,500 deaths per year – but it will cost only $195 million. It means that more people will develop, and die from, bladder cancer, but it will save some $250 million dollars that US taxpayers would have to pay every year to maintain the practice of water fluoridation.

George Glasser commented: 'The politicking over who will live and who will pay the ultimate price in the phoney war against tooth decay has to end.'

Arsenic in Irish fluoride

Every year, the Irish government pays hundreds of thousands of pounds to the Dutch company that produces the hexafluorosilicic acid used to fluoridate Irish drinking water. Until June 1996, the contract to supply fluorosilicic acid was held by Chemifloc Ltd., based in Shannon, Co. Clare. Their fluorosilicic acid is, they say, not derived from the waste of fertiliser production but is 'a manufactured product which is of high quality'.[4] However, the Eastern Health Board informed Chemifloc that, for reasons of cost, it had awarded the contract to another firm, Albatros Fertilizers of New Ross, Wexford. Albatros supply fertiliser-based waste from Holland. Chemifloc, in a letter to Dáil Éireann, the Irish parliament, pointed out that their fluorosilicic acid contained only 5–10 per cent of the arsenic content found in fertiliser-based products. They say in the letter: '[W]e did raise the issue of arsenic content with the Eastern Health Board but their attitude was that it met their specifications and it didn't matter if ours have substantially less arsenic.'

Health authorities that continued to use the Chemifloc

product ceased to do so in November 1996 'due to the intervention of Brendan Howlin, TD, Minister for the Environment, who told the local authorities they would only be able to recoup the cost of fluoridation if they purchased the material from Albatros'. Chemifloc asks: 'I wonder if the fact that Albatros is in Howlin's constituency influenced him?' They conclude: '[I]n any event you can be happy that not only is the Eastern Health Board ensuring that your water is fluoridated, they're also seeing you get a little extra arsenic at no charge. Personally I would prefer to do without the arsenic.'

In August 2000, Fluoride Free Water, the Irish campaign to free Ireland of the scourge of fluoride, had a sample of the fluorosilicic acid used in that country analysed.[5] This revealed an arsenic concentration of 4.826 ppm.

The silicon/cancer connection

Like fluorine, silicon is always found in nature compounded with other elements as a silicate. Silicon is not toxic in itself, but it is known to cause irritations in soft tissue, which can lead to the formation of cancers in the same way as asbestos fibres do. The *Merck Index*, an encyclopaedia of chemicals, drugs and biological agents, lists the amount of silica in H_2SiF_6 as 19.49 per cent.

Most silicon compounds that occur in nature are considered harmless, because silicon compounds are poorly absorbed. Nevertheless, silica derived from reacting fluorosilicic acid with lime is used to induce cancers in laboratory animals. While the silica itself is harmless, microscopic crystalline silica particles act as 'seeds' around which precancerous material forms.

The most damaging forms of silica – silicon halides and hydrides – are extremely toxic by either inhalation or ingestion. The most-used fluoridation agent both in Britain, Ireland and the US is hexafluorosilicic acid (H_2SiF_6), which, as chance would have it, is possibly the most easily metabolised silicon halide. Thus, almost everyone who drinks artificially fluoridated drinking water is exposed to this silicon halide.

George Glasser points out that each milligram of hexafluorosilicic acid that is put into drinking water 'releases millions of molecular fluorosilicate ions. Even if the fluorosilicate ion dissociates, as suggested by EPA and Centers for Disease Control (CDC) management, millions of silicon dioxide molecules remain as suspended solids. These submicroscopic silica molecules can be metabolised and circulated throughout soft tissues in the body. In contrast, EPA drinking water regulations only allow seven microscopic fibers of less than ten-millionths of a meter long in one liter of drinking water.'

On 10 May 1999, Ken Calvert, of the US House of Representatives' Subcommittee on Energy and the Environment, wrote to the US EPA asking what chronic toxicity test data there were on sodium fluorosilicate and hydrofluorosilicic acid. In a letter dated 23 June 1999, J. Charles Fox, an assistant administrator at EPA headquarters, answered that the EPA could find none.

Despite thousands of papers published both in Europe and America on silicon as a possible cause of cancer and Alzheimer's disease, silicon does not appear on Material Safety Data Sheets or in any quality-control specification sheets (contaminant analyses), and all government agencies refuse to acknowledge it.

George Glasser, an investigative journalist living in Florida, and Andreas Schuld investigated this oversight. One water-treatment quality-control laboratory, Underwriter's Laboratories, told them that they were not obliged to report silica/silicon levels. When Glasser and Schuld contacted the National Sanitation Foundation, the primary quality-control laboratory contracted by the US EPA, they received no response. Glasser and Schuld say: 'The avoidance of acknowledging the presence of silica/silicon in the water fluoridation agents is, more than likely, due to the fact that the fluorosilicates would have to be reclassified to no less than Group 2 substances (probable carcinogens). The reclassification would disrupt industry and put a halt to drinking water fluoridation. All drinking water fluoridation research papers would be worthless, and a whole new set of Federal regulations for occupational exposures would have to be drafted and implemented.'

Glasser and Schuld may not have got very far in their quest, but help is at hand. In May 2000, the US House of Representatives' Subcommittee on Energy and the Environment wrote again to the EPA, the National Academy of Sciences, the Centers for Disease Control and Prevention, the Food and Drugs Administration and manufacturer of silicofluorides NAS International, asking for specific test data that show that these substances are safe.

It does not matter whether the fluorosilicate radical dissociates or not: the mere presence of silica at a concentration of about 19 percent in the two chemicals allowed for water fluoridation is enough to classify them as carcinogens.

G proteins

While government agencies behave like ostriches, evidence of the dangers posed by silica continues to grow.

Since the first fluoridation experiments in the USA, knowledge about how our bodies react to environmental chemical influences has progressed. Many reports surfaced during the 1950s detailing how illnesses occurred faster and were more pronounced when fluorides were combined with silica. The subsequent discovery of G proteins, the molecular 'on/off' switches that control a wide range of biological processes such as protein synthesis, signal transduction pathways, cancer growth and cell differentiation, led to much greater understanding of a wide range of diseases from cancer to Alzheimer's disease.[6]

Damaged or mutated G-protein receptors are implicated in many diseases. Thousands of studies show how aluminium fluoride activates such G proteins to produce mutations in animal and human tissue. A further increase in these diseases can be expected, as silicon acts synergistically with fluoride. American government medical Web sites are replete with evidence of such information. The PubMed site, http://www. ncbi.nlm.nih.gov/entrez, offers more than 7,000 citations on silica or silicon. Cancerlit (http://cnetdb.nci.nih.gov/ cancerlit.shtml) and Grateful Med (http://igm.nlm.nih.gov/cgi) each offer several hundred citations on the association between silica/silicon exposures and cancers. There is no lack of evidence, and it is not difficult to find.

Brain tumours

Primary brain tumours are among the most deadly of all cancers, and rates are increasing worldwide at an alarming rate, especially among the elderly. Because of their location and the large numbers of different types of tumour that affect the brain, treatment by surgery is extremely difficult and hazardous.

In 1998 a statistically significant association was observed between the presence of brain tumours and the concentrations of silicon.[7] Although documented extensively in the European literature, the synergistic action of silicon and fluoride get scant attention by those who advocate fluoridation of water.

Conclusion

Despite the fact that H_2SiF_6 and other fluorosilicates are potentially carcinogenic, we are told that fluorosilicates will behave the same as sodium fluoride in any environment. Yet in more than fifty years of fluoridation, not one study has ever been conducted using the actual fluorosilicate compounds that are used in real life, to verify this statement. Thus, the possibility that long-term, low-level exposure to fluorosilicates in drinking water may cause cancer and other diseases is both untested and unknown.

Using the BFS's generic definition, any species of fluorides, no matter how toxic, carcinogenic or otherwise, could be substituted as a water fluoridation agent for the more benign, surrogate fluorides used for research purposes. We could even add sarin.

References

1. Kick CH et al. *Fluorine in animal nutrition.* Ohio Agricultural Experiment Station, Bulletin 558, November 1935: 61.

2. Roholm K. *Fluorine intoxication.* Copenhagen: Arnold Busck, 1937. Quoted in Waldbott GL. *A struggle with titans.* New York: Carlton Press, 1965: 79.

3. Glasser G. Fluoridation chemicals contain the highest levels of arsenci. http://home.att.net/~gtigerelaw/awwa/press.html.

4. Storey EA. Letter from Chemifloc Ltd. to Trevor Sargent, TD, 20 February 1997.

5. Chemical analysis, Confidential Report No. W8158, CAL Ltd., Dublin, 14 August 2000. http:/www.homepage.eircom.net/~fluoridefree/images/chemical_analysis.jpg.

6. Gilman AG. G proteins, transducers of receptor-generated signals. *Annu Rev Biochem* 1987; 56: 615–49.

7. Hadfield MG, Adera T, Smith B et al. Human brain tumours and exposure to metal and non-metal elements: a case-control study. *J Environ Pathol Toxicol Oncol* 1998; 17 (1): 1–9.

25. The History of Water Fluoridation, Part Two

Is it true that the fluoride used for fluoridation is toxic waste from the phosphate fertiliser industry, collected from the factory chimneys?

BFS suggested answer

It is not true. Fluoride used for water fluoridation is manufactured to very high quality standards which are set by the Department of Environment.

Two compounds of fluoride are permitted for artificial fluoridation in the UK: fluorosilicic acid (H_2SiF_6), and sodium fluorosilicate (Na_2SiF_6). These compounds are manufactured to exacting quality standards, and must meet Department of Environment purity specifications.

BFS suggested answer refuted

In regard to the use of fluosilicic [fluorosilicic] acid as a source of fluoride for fluoridation, this agency regards such use as an ideal environmental solution to a long-standing problem. By recovering by-product fluosilicic acid from fertilizer manufacturing, water and air pollution are minimized, and water utilities have a low-cost source of fluoride available to the communities.
Official US EPA policy, 1983

The marketing of fluoride in the USA continued apace as fluoride waste was produced in ever greater quantities. In a 1983 letter from the Environmental Protection Agency, then deputy assistant administrator in the Office for Water,

Rebecca Hamner, wrote the quotation above.[1] She aims to reduce (air) pollution by increasing (water) pollution!

Today, about 130 million Americans in 9,600 communities drink fluoridated water.[2] But the fluoridation agent is no longer sodium fluoride. That became too expensive when a cheaper source of fluoride was found.

Fertiliser industries' waste replaces metal industries' waste

The aluminium industry was not the only industry with concerns about how to minimise the cost of getting rid of their toxic fluoride wastes. In the 1940s the Blockson Chemical Company of Joliet, Illinois, sponsored a year-long survey 'to develop new uses for sodium fluosilicate', the waste product of the phosphate fertiliser industry.[3] Almost all of the sodium fluorosilicate produced today is a by-product of the phosphate industry and is derived from the calcium fluoride and fluorapatite in phosphate rock.

In 1931 Frank McClure wrote a PhD thesis about the toxic effects of fluoride contained in rock phosphate.[4] In 1943 he wrote again of fluoride's toxicity: 'The production of endemic dental fluorosis in human beings by fluoride in drinking water is an outstanding example of the toxic effect of an excessive intake of the element.'[5] Despite this, in 1950 McClure looked at the possibility of using sodium fluorosilicate in place of sodium fluoride for water fluoridation.[6]

Certainly, other chemicals were needed if fluoridation of the USA was to be continued and extended. Sodium fluoride was becoming scarce. Sodium fluorosilicate looked like the answer. However, its production too needed to be stepped up if fluoridation was to expand. In August 1951 the American Office of Price Stabilization granted higher price ceilings to manufacturers of sodium silicofluoride to promote its manufacture and add impetus to the fluoridation programme.[7]

In the USA today, practically all of the fluorosilicates used for water fluoridation come from the phosphate fertiliser industry in Florida.

The origins of the product

During the process of manufacturing phosphoric acid from phosphate-rich rock, several chemicals are added, and inherent toxic contaminants common in phosphate rock are boiled off. These vapours are classified as 'hazardous air pollutants'. Their release into the atmosphere is prohibited. Thus, chimneys of phosphate plants are fitted with 'scrubbers' to wash the emitted gases and capture these pollutant chemicals. The scrubbing process removes not just the fluorides but all pollutants, including pollution from tank farms and other processes. The more efficient the scrubbing operation, the more contaminants will be concentrated in the scrubber liquor. The resultant pollution is a toxic liquid that contains a mixture of all the chemicals scrubbed from the waste gases.

Phosphoric acid reaction vessels are made of the alloy Hastelloy G-30. These vessels are corroded by the presence of fluorides and chlorides in the phosphoric acid and last on average three years. The metals from Hastelloy G-30, which include cancer-causing nickel and beryllium, are also present in the fluorosilicic acid as metal-complexed fluorosilicates.

Sulphuric acid is produced at these facilities, and the spent vanadium pentoxide catalyst, production sludge and waste water are dumped into the evaporation (settling) ponds, the catch-all for almost all toxic wastes. Radioactive scale from reaction vessels and filters, phosphoric acid sludges, radioactive fluorosilicates chipped from scrubbing pads and chambers, and general toxic wastes are also tossed into the mix.

To make matters worse, evaporation-pond water is always used in the pollution scrubbers because there are strict regulations regarding fresh water usage in Florida. Most of the waste water, sludges and waste chemicals from the analytical laboratories are dumped into the evaporation ponds, which are reused in the production of fluorosilicic acid for water fluoridation.

By now it should be evident that we are not dealing with a simple, pure, reagent-grade fluorosilicic acid purchased from a chemical supply house, as the BFS would have us believe. Even if the product had no fluorides present, it would be dangerous to put in the water, but with the complex chemical reactions and possible reactions with both organic and inorganic compounds, the fluoridating product is potentially extremely toxic.

The most frightening aspect is that no two batches are the same, and the toxic effects can vary from batch to batch. There will also be a variance from company to company supplying the product, because of the types and grades of chemicals, quality of the phosphate rock, processes and kind of solvent extraction method used to produce phosphoric acid.

Do they think we're stupid?

In 2000, Jane Jones, campaign director of the National Pure Water Association, attempted to find safety test data – any evidence at all – that would support the safety of the fluorosilicate products. She wrote repeatedly to dental spokespersons in the USA and the World Health Organization, and to US fluoridation engineers. Not one could quote a single study in its support. In fact, they refused to answer. There can be no doubt that there is something decidedly fishy about this product.

Jane Jones's requests for safety data and George Glasser's articles really hit a nerve: there was a great deal of consternation in the pro-fluoride camp, particularly about the use of the term 'pollution scrubbers'. During a bitterly fought campaign to prevent fluoridation in Wellington, Florida, the Palm Beach

County dental director, Robert Dumbaugh, wrote to the director of environmental health, Frank Gargiulo, seeking help:[8]

> Frank
>
> You can see what we are up against. This argument represents the major thrust of the opposition in Wellington. We will have to come up with some very convincing explanation that defuses the mass hysteria surrounding 'pollution scrubbers' and toxic waste dumping. Any suggestions? They even have Tom Reeves on the ropes now. I think we have to have somebody that understands the industrial process and can speak to the regulations which govern and permit the production of fluorosilicic acid, and speak to the safety issue.
>
> Thanks
>
> Bob

For the next couple of months e-mails hurtled through the ether asking if anyone could come up with a solution and a counter to the derogatory term 'pollution scrubber'. Not an easy task when you consider that 'pollution scrubber' is the exact phrase the industry gives to the process used to remove fluoride pollution. How could the champions of fluoride refute it?

Well, it seems 'pollution' isn't pollution if it doesn't reach the environment (mind you, it does reach the environment when it is put in tap water, but let's disregard that for now). As the scrubbers stop the silicofluorides from being vented to the atmosphere, these silicofluorides are no longer 'pollution'.

Distinguished EPA scientist Dr William Hirzy, as previously noted, poured scorn on this obvious attempt to manipulate the facts, saying: '[I]f this stuff gets out into the air, it's a pollutant; if it gets into the river, it's a pollutant; if it gets into the lake, it's a pollutant; but if it goes right straight into your drinking water system, it's not a pollutant. That's amazing!'[9]

Now, the pro-fluoride camp had to get rid of that other obnoxious word 'scrubber'. The following e-mail from Tom Reeves, national fluoridation engineer, USPHS, was sent to explain how it could be done:

Hi Folks,

There is a small point of correction I would like to make about the production of the fluorosilicic acid. A lot of people sometimes say, even once in a while myself, that the acid is captured with pollution scrubbers. That is not technically correct.

As most of you know, the apatite rock is ground up and treated with sulfuric acid, forming a gas by-product. The fluorosilicic acid is evaporated off the phosphoric acid and captured as fluorosilicic acid using fresh water and is condensed into a lined recycle system. These units are called product recovery units. The fluorosilicic acid does not come from pollution scrubbers and is not vented into the air. Pollution scrubbers usually do not use fresh, very clean, water. This is a small point because the pollution scrubbers and the product recovery units are similar. But since the antis make such a big point about the 'pollution' part of the pollution scrubbers, maybe we should start using the correct term.

I have said for many years that the impurities in the apatite is [sic] lead, arsenic and zinc. Chuck Krepshaw of Cargill Fertilizer Inc., the producer of about 70–75% of the F chemicals used in the US, tells me now that in the newer vein of apatite rock, the impurities are very small amounts of lead, arsenic, mercury and barium. Of course when diluted into water, contain amounts that would all be much less than a part per billion, and in most cases, would be undetectable in fluoridated water without the use of highly specialized equipment.

I hope this clarifies this issue.

TOM

And with that sorted out, 'toxic waste' could become 'beneficial nutrient'.

Conclusion

The products used for water fluoridation for decades are waste from the manufacture of phosphate fertiliser. They are a 'soup' of impurities on which no safety testing has ever been done. Scientists have drawn attention to the fact that the only other place this fluorosilicic acid can legally be disposed of is in a hazardous waste facility.

Vendors selling the pollution concentrate as a fluoridation agent use a broad disclaimer found on the Material Data Safety Sheet:

> [N]o responsibility can be assumed by vendor for any damage or injury resulting from abnormal use, from any failure to adhere to recommended practices, **or from any hazards inherent to the product.** [Emphasis added]

In other words, you drink fluoridated water at your own risk.

References

1. Rebecca Hanmer, deputy administrator, Office of Water, US EPA. Correspondence with Dr Leslie Russell stating US EPA position on water fluoridation, 1983. Quoted in Glasser G. *Fluoride in the drinking water: It's pollution, stupid!* 1 February 2000. http://www.npwa.freeserve.co.uk/pollution.htm.
2. Hileman B. Fluoridation of Water. *Chem Eng News* 1988; 29; Brunelle JA, Carlos JP. Recent trends in dental caries in US children and the effect of water fluoridation. *J Dent Res.* 1990; 69: 723–7.
3. Hampel CA. Sodium fluosilicate – a neglected chemical. *Chem Eng News* 1949; 27: 2420.

4. McClure FJ, Mitchell HH. The effect of fluorine on the calcium metabolism of albino rats and the compostion of the bones. *J Biol Chem* 1931; 90: 297–320.
5. McClure FJ. Ingestion of fluoride and dental caries – quantitative relations based on food and water requirements of children 1 to 12 years old. *Am J Dis Child* 1943; 66: 362.
6. McClure FJ. Availability of fluorine in sodium fluoride vs. sodium fluosilicate. *Public Health Rep* 1950; 65: 1175.
7. Water fluoridation. *J Am Dent Assoc* 1951; 43: 499–500.
8. Glasser G. Fluoridation findings set teeth gnashing. http://www.npa.freeserve.co.uk/pants_down_comments .html.
9. Hirzy JW. Video interview with Michael Connett. 3 July 2000. Unpublished.

26. Dentifrice – or Rodenticide?

Is it the same fluoride that is used as rat poison?

BFS suggested answer
No. Fluoride in water is not a poison, it is safe and beneficial.

BFS suggested answer refuted
Neither will I administer a poison to anybody when asked to do so, nor will I suggest such a course.
The Hippocratic Oath

Sodium fluoride was the first compound used to fluoridate public water systems artificially. It caused an uproar because sodium fluoride was a poison used commercially as an insecticide, rodenticide, wood preservative and fungicide.[1] The US federal government clearly recognised the toxicity of sodium fluoride: as an active ingredient in pesticides, the Federal Insecticide, Fungicide, and Rodenticide Act[2] required the prominent display on the container of a skull-and-crossbones symbol and the word 'Poison'.[3]

Government promoters seeking to add fluoride to the public water systems back in the 1950s held a conference and attempted to defuse this issue by instructing those in attendance not to use the word 'artificial' in conjunction with fluoridation, and not to tell the public that sodium fluoride was being used, because 'that is rat poison'.[4] Instead, the public should be told only that 'fluorides' are added to the water.

Sodium fluoride is not used in Britain or Ireland for the fluoridation of tap water. But it is still used extensively in toothpastes, gels, mouthwashes and other dental products – check the labels!

Sodium fluoride and stomach haemorrhages

Sodium fluoride (NaF) or sodium monofluorophosphate (MFP) is put in toothpaste and other dental preparations. In 1992 a randomised double-blind study was published in which healthy male volunteers were given either sodium fluoride or sodium monofluorophosphate tablets for just seven days. Before the trial began, the linings of their stomachs were evaluated. On the first day of the trial and at the end of the week, the linings of their stomachs were examined again and compared. At the same times, blood fluoride values were measured. Throughout the trial, blood fluoride levels were similar in both treatment groups, but this was not the case with their stomachs. Examination of these disclosed significant differences between the two groups. In the MFP group, the researchers found nothing out of the ordinary, but in the NaF group seven of the ten subjects had significant stomach lesions, including acute haemorrhages and free blood in their stomachs. There were also four times as many possible adverse drug reactions in the NaF group compared with the MFP group. Summing up, the study's authors, Dr P. Muller and colleagues, say: '[U]nder the experimental conditions used MFP is well tolerated by the stomach while NaF produces significant gastric mucosal lesions.'[5]

Fluoride supplements aren't safe either

In 1992, New Jersey assemblyman, John V. Kelly, was concerned when he read of Cohn's cancer studies in that state. He immediately contacted the American Academy of Pediatric Dentistry and asked them to send him studies supporting the safety and effectiveness of fluoride supplements that also contain sodium fluoride.

The Academy promised to send them, but, he says, they never came. When he pressed the Academy members, they admitted that they had no such studies but informed him the studies could be obtained from the National Institute of Dental Research. Again, no studies were forthcoming, and the NIDR respondents admitted that they had no studies. They suggested that Kelly go straight to the Food and Drugs Administration (FDA), since that agency was responsible for approving these products. He waited six months and was 'stunned when I was advised by the FDA that **fluoride supplements were not approved by the FDA** [emphasis in original]. Incredibly, in fifty years, no one has ever bothered submitting a petition to the FDA to have these products approved!' He continued:

> It is my understanding that in 1975, the FDA issued a regulatory letter asking manufacturers to remove fluoride supplements from the market. To date, the FDA has not responded to my inquiry asking for clarification of their actions in 1975. Also, in 1993 I petitioned the FDA to enforce the law and remove children's fluoride supplements from the market. The FDA has ignored my repeated requests.

On 14 August 2000, Kelly wrote to Senator Robert Smith, chairman of the Environment and Public Works Committee, Washington, DC, telling him of his findings on the lack of safety studies for dental supplements.[6] 'At best,' he wrote,

> fluoride supplements are a waste of precious health care dollars. At worst, they are causing real harm to our infants and children.
>
> I urge you to hold hearings on this issue. I also urge you to demand that the FDA enforce the law and remove these unapproved products from the market.

Conclusion

The duplicity of the BFS's answer is exposed if we compare it to the answer in Chapter 24. In that, the BFS avers that fluoride is the same no matter what it is compounded with, yet in answer to this question says that this fluoride is not the same.

References

1. *Safe Water Association, Inc.* v. *City of Fond Du Lac,* 516 N.W.2d 13, 17 (Wis. Ct. App. 1994), review dismissed, 520 N.W.2d 91, Wisconsin, 1994.

2. FIFRA requires the registration of all new pesticides, as well as the reregistration of pesticides first registered before 1 November 1984. See Federal Insecticide, Fungicide, and Rodenticide Act, 7 USC §§ 136a, 136a-1 (1991) (exceptions omitted). The Special Review and Reregistration Division in the EPA's Office of Pesticide Programs publishes a document called the *Rainbow report* (Status of Pesticides in Reregistration and Special Review), which lists sodium fluoride as an active ingredient in pesticides. See Environmental Protection Agency, *Pesticide active ingredients index.* Sodium fluoride was originally labelled as an 'economic poison' under FIFRA. See 7 USC § 135a(a)(4) (1981). 'The term "economic poison" means (1) any substance or mixture of substances intended for preventing, destroying, repelling, or mitigating any insects, rodents, nematodes, fungi, weeds, and other forms of plant or animal life or viruses, except viruses on or in living man or other animals, which the Administrator shall declare to be a pest . . .' 7 USC § 135(a).

3. See 7 USC § 136(q)(2)(D), 1991.

4. Statement of Dr John W. Knutson, chief, Division of Dental Public Health, at the Proceedings of the Fourth Annual Conference of State Dental Directors with the Public Health Service and the Children's Bureau, Federal Security Building, Washington, DC, USA, 6–8 June 1951. See also: *Promotion and application of water fluoridation: Hearings before the Dept of Labor and Health, Education and Welfare Appropriations*, 89th Congress, Vol. 5, 1967.

5. Muller P, Schmid K, Warnecke G, Setniker I, Simon B. Sodium fluoride-induced gastric mucosal lesions: comparison with sodium monofluorophosphate. *Gastroenterology* 1992; 30: 252–4.

6. Kelly JV. Letter to Senator Robert Smith, chairman, Environment and Public Works Committee, Washington, DC, 14 August 2000.

27. Europe Against Fluoride

> ## Why has fluoridation been banned in several European countries?
>
> ### BFS suggested answer
>
> Fluoridation has not been banned anywhere. Over 300 million people world-wide drink fluoridated water – including over half the population of the USA.
>
> *Some European countries which have discontinued water fluoridation, such as the Netherlands and Finland, have done so for political reasons, NOT BECAUSE OF FEAR OF ADVERSE HEALTH EFFECTS.*
>
> *Fluoride toothpastes are widely used throughout Europe, and most countries use other forms of fluoride delivery to prevent tooth decay. For example, Ireland, the UK and Spain have extensive water fluoridation. Elsewhere, salt is fluoridated, e.g. France, Germany, Belgium and Switzerland.*
>
> ### BFS suggested answer refuted
>
> *Most of the world has rejected fluoridation. Only America where it originated, and countries under strong American influence persist in the practice.*
>
> Dr John Colquhoun, former chief dental officer, Auckland, NZ

Fluoridation is far less widely accepted than its proponents would have us believe. Fluoridation has been strongly opposed throughout the world. Today, only five countries worldwide – all English-speaking – fluoridate to any large extent. At the top of the fluoridation league are Ireland at about 75 per cent and Australia at 66 per cent fluoridated; the USA, Canada and New Zealand tie for third place on 50 percent. England is a lowly sixth at less than 10 per cent – which is hardly 'extensive'. This is because the dangers of fluoridation have not gone unnoticed. In western continental Europe, fluoridation has been a total flop. The fact is that only about 2 per cent of the people of Western Europe today drink fluoridated water, almost all of them within the British Isles.

Austria

According to M. Eisenhut, head of the Water Department, Österreichische Vereinigung für das Gas- und Wasserfach, '[T]oxic fluorides have never been added to the public water supplies in Austria.'[1]

Germany

Fluoridation was introduced experimentally in the West German town of Kassel in 1952. After two years, Germany rejected fluoridation because the recommended dosage of 1 ppm was 'too close to the dose at which long-term damage to the human body is to be expected'.

Parts of the former East Germany were fluoridated from 1959 until reunification in 1990. Drs W. Künzel and T. Fischer analysed the dental records of more than 286,000 subjects of both sexes (six to fifteen years old) from two industrial towns: Chemnitz (formerly Karl-Marx-Stadt), which was fluoridated from 1959 to 1990, with a 22-month interruption around 1971, and Plauen, 75 per cent fluoridated from 1972 to 1984.[2] Water fluoridation was followed by a decrease of caries, and interruptions in fluoridation were followed by increasing caries levels. However, after German reunification, a different caries trend was observed. Between the years 1987 and 1995, instead of an expected rise in dental decay, there was a significant decrease down to the lowest DMFT (2.0) since 1959, despite fluoridation having ceased in the two cities. Today, all of Germany is unfluoridated.[3]

Luxembourg

'Fluoride has never been added to the public water supplies in Luxembourg. In our views, the drinking water isn't the suitable way for medicinal treatment and that people needing an addition of fluoride can decide by their own to use the most appropriate way, like the intake of fluoride tablets, to cover their daily needs.'[4]

Denmark

According to the Danish Ministry of Environment and Energy, 'toxic fluorides have never been added to the public water supplies in Denmark. Consequently, no Danish city has ever been fluoridated.'[5] After fluoridation of water was first mooted in Denmark, on 3 January 1977, the National Agency of Environmental Protection recommended that the Minister not permit fluoridation. This recommendation was based upon the fact that a number of questions concerning human health and the environment were not and could not be clarified. In his answer to a question from the Committee on Fluoridation of Drinking Water, on 5 January 1977, the Danish Minister for the Environment, Helge Nielsen, stated that in his opinion the power conferred by Section 48 of the Water Supply Act should not be used to allow the addition of fluoride to drinking water. His reasons were that no adequate studies had been carried out on its long-term effects on human organ systems other than teeth, and that not enough studies had been done on the effect of fluoride discharges on freshwater ecosystems. The Ministry of the Interior issued a public announcement: '[F]luoridation of public water supplies as well as of all consumables is prohibited.' Denmark also banned fluoride supplements in January 1964.

Finland

Kuopio is a city that features prominently in medical journals and medical trials. Drs Helmer Nordling and Inkeri Tulikoura conducted a study there between 1958, when it was first fluoridated, and 1968, with Jyväskylä as the control city. Their results were published in 1970.[6] The study continued until 1984 and showed the importance of continuing studies over a long period of time. By 1968, 7-year-old children in fluoridated Kuopio had 55 per cent fewer cavities than in unfluoridated Jyväskylä. This looked like a good result, but four years later the difference between the two cities was down to 46 percent. By 1975 it had reduced to 19 percent, and by 1976 the cavity rates in both cities were identical. In 1990 fluoridation was stopped in Kuopio because of fears about osteoporosis. In 1998, Dr L. Seppa and colleagues published a study that examined the consequences of this discontinuation on dental health.[7] Despite the children not having fluoridated water any more, Seppa and colleagues found no sign of an increasing trend in dental decay. They also found that other fluoride dental treatments were useless; their findings suggested 'that the decline of caries has little to do with professional preventive measures performed in dental clinics'. There is now no fluoridation in Finland.

Norway

There was a rather intense discussion about fluoridation in Norway around 1980. The conclusion was that drinking water should not be fluoridated. The decision was taken that it was up to each individual to decide whether to use fluoride in tablets, toothpaste or mouthwash to prevent caries. There is now no ongoing political discussion in Norway concerning fluoridation of drinking water. Norway remains unfluoridated.[8]

Sweden

In 1961 Sweden's Supreme Court declared that fluoridation was illegal. Nevertheless, in 1969 Professor Yngve Ericsson, a Swedish dentist, and the senior representative on the World Health Organization's Expert Committee on Fluoridation, strongly advised the Swedes to fluoridate their water supply. It was then found that Professor Ericsson was the holder of two highly profitable patents on fluoride toothpaste; and a subsequent investigation disclosed that the WHO's numerous so-called 'objective' comparative studies on mortality and morbidity for fluoridated vs. unfluoridated areas simply didn't exist. The investigation stated that the WHO's report was unacceptable from a scientific point of view; that some of the claims set forth in the WHO report actually lacked any and every basis in fact; and that the details given by WHO on risks and safety margins were grossly defective. Sweden's Nobel Medical Institute, after conducting a ten-year study, recommended against fluoridation. In 1971 the Swedish parliament repealed the country's fluoridation law, stating: '[V]alid evidence to support the claims widely quoted by fluoridation proponents simply does not exist.' Fluoridation was banned in 1972.[9]

The Netherlands

Tiel was the first city to be fluoridated in 1953. It was included in a trial of the effects of fluoridation on dental cavities with Culemborg as the control city. These two cities were not chosen at random. In 1949, a young dentist named Joseph Fick had researched the decay-causing properties of yoghurt. He found that an extracted tooth placed in yoghurt started to decay after two days, and after a week there was a cavity. In his study, he compared the children of Culemborg and Tiel, noting that the children of Culemborg ate twice as much yoghurt as the children of Tiel. They also had twice as much dental decay. As it was known that cavity rates between the two cities were so different, it was not a fair trial.

In 1970, Dr Hans Moolenburgh, a doctor whose practice spanned the Dutch towns of Haarlem and Heemstede, a suburb of Amsterdam, noticed that after Amsterdam was fluoridated, patients from the now-fluoridated Heemstede began to suffer a variety of mysterious diseases, whereas no change was seen in illness patterns in unfluoridated Haarlem. Reasoning that fluoride might be to blame, Moolenburgh carried out the only double-blind trial ever to have been conducted into the effects of fluoride, and proved beyond doubt that fluoride was the cause. Over the next six years he, joined by others, amassed a vast body of evidence against fluoride.[10]

On 22 June 1973, the Dutch Supreme Court ruled that there was no legal basis for fluoridation.[11] After that judgement, an amendment to the Water Supply Act was prepared to provide a legal basis for fluoridation, despite the fact that there was a swelling tide of opinion in the Dutch parliament against it.

On 9 March 1976, the Dutch Minister of Health, Irene Vorrink, introduced a bill to fluoridate all of Holland. The next day came confirmation from the American National Cancer Institute that they had observed a rise in cancer deaths. Moolenburgh sent it directly to parliament.

Parliamentary discussions had centred not on the harm that fluoride could do but on the question of personal freedom and how the government could make provision to supply unfluoridated water to those who did not wish to drink fluoridated tap water. On 16 March, Health Minister Vorrink suggested: 'Let us keep these provisions for those who object outside this bill. There is already one easy solution, namely a filter on your tap. Experts are busy developing such a filter.' The Dutch parliament was adjourned while someone tried to find out about this filter. But nobody knew anything about such a filter. The Dutch press had a field day.

As the result of Moolenburgh's work, the Dutch rewrote their constitution to ensure that the practice of fluoridation would never be allowed in that country again.

Switzerland[12]

Basle was fluoridated in 1962. Children of the city, aged between seven and fifteen, were examined at five-year intervals. There was no attempt to use a control group, thus this could show neither benefit nor harm in any scientifically acceptable way. However, had there been a reduction in caries, a reduction in the number of dentists needed might have demonstrated the fact. But while there were only ten dentists practising in Basle in 1960, eight years later that number had almost doubled. It is not surprising, therefore, that the Swiss Department of Health suggested in 1975 that fluoridation in Basle should cease, as it had failed to reduce tooth decay.

France

France has never fluoridated its populace. France's universally respected Pasteur Institute and Sweden's Nobel Institute agree that fluoride has little or no value as a dental cavity deterrent and stress that health risks from using fluoride outweigh any benefits. After consulting with the Pasteur Institute, France's chief counsel of public health rejected fluoridation in 1980 because of possible harm to human health.

Italy and Belgium

Italy and Belgium, like France, rejected fluoridation outright.

Spain

Parts of Spain may be fluoridated. There appears to be a cover-up there, and nobody seems to know what the true picture is. The last official figure I saw was that 3 per cent of Spanish water supplies were fluoridated, but that figure may be higher now. So far as I can ascertain, Seville, Granada, Murcia and some northern cities are fluoridated, and the provinces of Andalusia, Navarra and the Basque Country have decided to fluoridate their water supplies. There is a factory in Bilbao, apparently state-owned, called Derivados del Fluor, which may be the source of the fluoride.[13] But if Spain is fluoridated, it is not helping its children's teeth, as Spain is well down the WHO cavity league table.

Hungary

In the early 1960s, one city, Szolnok, was fluoridated, but fluoridation was very soon stopped for technical reasons. Since that date, despite significant technological advances that could have allowed fluoridation to recommence, Hungary remains unfluoridated.[14]

Portugal and Greece

These two countries experimented with fluoride and then abandoned it.

Ireland

Water fluoridation was introduced into Ireland in 1964. Ireland is unique in the world now as the only democratic country where fluoridation is mandatory by law. Even the USA hasn't dared to go that far. Two-thirds or more of the population have had fluoridated water since its inception, yet as we saw in Chapter 1, WHO figures, showing Ireland lying in a lowly sixth place behind unfluoridated countries, do not support the claim that fluoridation of drinking water helps to preserve Irish children's teeth.

In May 2000 Irish Minister for Health, Micheál Martin, announced the formation of a Forum on Fluoridation, similar to the UK Review (see Chapter 33), 'to review the fluoridation of public piped water supplies', because of the public's growing concerns about fluoride.[15]

The Forum was to have had representatives from consumer and environmental groups, but one, Darina Allen, refused to be involved when she saw the pro-fluoridation bias of the panel, and another, Dick Warner, said he had never agreed to have his name put forward in the first place.

Not unreasonably, Éamon Gilmore, TD, Labour Party Environment spokesman, warned the Minister: 'Pending the outcome of this forum, there should be an embargo on the fluoridation of any new water schemes which may come on stream in the interim.'[16] However, like Britain, fluoridation will continue in Ireland while this 'Forum' meets, and, moreover, despite the public's resentment at being forced to drink fluoride-contaminated water, plans are in hand to fluoridate even more areas of the country before the Forum reports.

Fluoride Free Water, an Irish anti-fluoride organisation, says it 'has no longer any confidence in the "Forum on Fluoridation"', calling it a 'Fluoride Fiasco' and a 'cynical political ploy'.[17]

But all that may change. In January 2001, Fine Gael's Environment spokesman, Ivan Yates, said: 'Fine Gael believes that there are sufficient grounds to point to serious health risks from the cumulative amount of fluoride in our piped water supply system.' If elected, he pledged, the party would move both to end fluoridation because of 'serious health concerns' and to order every health board to investigate existing levels of fluoride in groundwater supplies.[18]

Fluoridated salt

As the BFS says, in some countries – France, Germany, Belgium and Switzerland – salt is fluoridated instead of water.[19] This is more consumer-friendly, as it does at least give consumers the choice of whether they want to ingest fluoride or not. But note that teeth in countries that fluoridate salt, just like those in countries that fluoridate water, are well down the European DMFT league tables.

Other countries

Japan

Influenced by America, Japan fluoridated its water supplies after World War II. But research soon showed the harm that fluoride could do. The Japanese were worried about the impact of fluoridated water on human health. As a consequence, Japan reduced the maximum amount of fluoride allowed in drinking water to one-eighth of that in the USA, and allowed only natural calcium fluoride to be added even then. As individuals differ, the Japanese feel that fluoridation is an inappropriate application that may cause health problems to vulnerable people and that there are better ways of protecting their people's dental health.[20] Japan is not fluoridated.

China

Gao Xishui, in a letter from the Ministry of Health, People's Republic of China, states: '[H]aving consulted with the Ministry of Construction we would like to inform you that it is not allowed to add fluoride into public drinking water in accordance with the regulations of the *Hygiene Standards of Public Drinking Water in China.*'[21]

Australia

Some of Australia's fluoride laws are so draconian that people can be prosecuted for speaking out against water fluoridation.[22]

There was so much disquiet in Australia about fluoride that in 1989 a law was passed in New South Wales to prohibit town councils from stopping the fluoridation of their water supplies without the permission of the health department.

In November 1994, just as the parliament of Victoria was about to rise for the summer recess, its members passed an amendment to the Fluoridation Act to change the constitution of Victoria in order to stop the Supreme Court of Victoria from hearing any cases or evidence against fluoridation. In support of the change, the Health Minister of Victoria said the alteration to the constitution had been made because 'fluoridation is important'. Not one member asked: 'What does the Minister mean by important?' On 28 December, Dr W.G. Hart, manager of health protection, Public Health Branch, wrote officially in a letter:

> With respect to compensation the Department does not accept liability for alleged damage caused by water fluoridation and will not support any claims for compensation.

The following year, the Tasmanian government went one step further by passing a bill through the Lower House to prohibit the holding of meetings on the subject of fluoridation. Called the Consequential Amendments Bill, this prohibited the discussion of fluoridation in private, public, councils, legal parties, schools where education is supposed to be provided, indeed anywhere in Tasmania. This was based on a special clause declaring fluoridation of public drinking water supplies to be an 'issue of significant interest'.

It certainly is!

Later, the Tasmanian bill was withdrawn to be reworded and reissued at a later date.

Conclusion

Throughout Europe, and in the rest of the world, wherever it is possible to discuss and debate water fluoridation, the process is banned, has been abandoned, or has never been adopted in the first place. It is only in countries in which the law makes fluoridation mandatory, or discussion of fluoridation illegal, that fluoride is widely used.

Fluoridation is the longest, most expensive and most spectacularly unsuccessful marketing campaign ever to come out of the United States.

References

1. Letter from M. Eisenhut, Österreichische Vereinigung für das Gas- und Wasserfach, Vienna, 17 February 2000.

2. Künzel W, Fischer T. Rise and fall of caries prevalence in German towns with different F concentrations in drinking water. *Caries Res* 1997; 31: 166–73.

3. Letter from Bundesministerium für Gesundheit, Bonn, 11 February 2000.

4. Ries J-M. Head, Water Department, Administration de L'Environnement, Luxembourg, 3 May 2000.

5. Letter from Royal Danish Embassy, Washington, DC, 22 December 1999.

6. Nordling H, Tulikoura I. *Finlands Tandläkartinding* 1970; 17 (11): 517.

7. Seppa L, Karkkainen S, Hausen H. Caries frequency in permanent teeth before and after discontinuation of water fluoridation in Kuopio, Finland. *Community Dent Oral Epidemiol* 1998; 26: 256–62.

8. Letter from National Institute of Public Health, Oslo, 1 March 2000.

9. *Gothenburg Post* (Sweden), 13 June 1970; *News Register* (Sweden), 5 Aug 1970; *Norsk Folkehelselag*

(Norway), 1 May 1970; Caldwell G. *Fluoridation and truth decay*. Top-Ecol Press, Reseda, California. 1974: 287.

10. Moolenburgh H. *Fluoride*: *The freedom fight*. Edinburgh: Mainstream Publishing, 1987.

11. *Budding and Co. v. City of Amsterdam*. Case No: 10683.

12. For data on most countries see letters to Mr E Albright of New Versailles, PA, USA from various officials in those countries. Can be accessed at http://www.fluoridealert.org *or* http://www.fluoridation.com.

13. Fluoridation in Spain. International Fluoride Information Network, 14 Feb 2000. http://www.fluoridealert.org/1fin-47.htm.

14. Letter from Ministry for Environment, Department for International Relations, Republic of Hungary, 24 January 2000.

15. Irish Department of Health press release, 29 May 2000.

16. Éamon Gilmore, TD. Statement, Monday, 29 May 2000.

17. http://homepage.eircom.net/~fluoridefree/CampaignUpdate/PressRelease111000.htm. Accessed 21 October 2000.

18. FG election promise to ban fluoride in drinking water. *Irish Independent* online, 15 January 2001. http://www.independent.ie/2001/14/n03e.shtml. Accessed 15 January 2001.

19 WHO Oral Health Country/Area Profile Programme, Dept. of Noncommunicable Diseases Surveillance/Oral Health. WHO Collaborating Centre, Malmö University, Sweden.

20 Letter from Toru Nagayama, Environment Agency, Tokyo, Japan, 8 March 2000.

21 Letter from Ministry of Health, People's Republic of China, 1 March 2000.

22. Living in a democratic fluoridated country. *Australian Fluoridation News* September–October 1995; 31 (5).

28. Skeletal Fluorosis

Is it true that in India fluoride in water causes severe skeletal deformity due to skeletal fluorosis?

BFS suggested answer

The situation in the UK is *completely* different from that in remote villages in India. Low levels of fluoride in drinking water in Birmingham and Newcastle have brought *huge* health benefits in terms of a *massive reduction in tooth decay* for *millions* of children for over 30 years.

The safety of low levels of fluoride in drinking water is endorsed by the World Health Organization, the British Medical Association, the British Dental Association and the Royal College of Physicians.

A Guardian article published in July 1995 describes severe skeletal deformity of the limbs of children living in a village in Central India.

Drinking water for the village was heavily contaminated with unsafe levels of natural chemicals including fluoride, arsenic, iron and salts.

The article also claimed that 17% of the population of another village near Delhi, where the drinking water contained between 0.7 and 1.6 ppm, suffered from skeletal fluorosis.

Skeletal fluorosis is undoubtedly a serious problem in parts of India and Pakistan. However, in temperate climates, such as the UK, USA and Canada, there is no evidence that skeletal fluorosis occurs – even in populations where the level of fluoride in drinking water is far in excess of those seen in the UK.

Dr AK Susheela, who was featured in the Guardian article, has visited the UK to campaign against fluoridation with the National Pure Water Association.

BFS suggested answer refuted
When medical practitioners everywhere also recognize the severity of the problems of chronic fluoride toxicosis, and laws mandating truly safe drinking water are sincerely enforced, the health of millions will dramatically improve.
Dr George L. Waldbott

Get rid of fluoride

In the 1970s and 1980s UN organisations tried very hard to promote water fluoridation in India despite the fact that it was already well known that there were prevailing health problems due to an excess of fluoride. Millions of people in sixteen Indian states are afflicted with skeletal fluorosis, leading to severe conditions such as malformed spine, neck and pelvis, weakened tooth structure and mottled or discoloured teeth. As a consequence, scientific studies of fluoridated water have been performed much more thoroughly in India than in the West. Dr A.K. Susheela of the India Institute of Medical Sciences in New Delhi found that, contrary to what the BFS would have us believe, fluoride severely disrupts the formation of the bone matrix, thereby inhibiting the proper hardening of bones.

According to Susheela, there are twenty nations in the world with serious health problems due to excess fluoride ingestion. They include India, China, and parts of Thailand and Africa; Japan, New Zealand, Australia, Israel, Pakistan, Syria and Turkey are also severely affected; and the problem also exists in Britain, the USA and Canada to a lesser extent. In the Western countries, better nutrition, with more calcium and Vitamin C in the diet, tends to nullify the toxic manifestations to some extent.[1]

Dr Susheela's work showing that high levels of fluoride in drinking water were clearly associated with birth defects, stillbirths and early infant mortality was so stunning and conclusive that in 1986 it prompted the Indian government to authorise the construction of *defluoridation* plants for drinking water. Intense scientific debates helped the Indian government in 1992 to amend the Drugs and Cosmetics Act of 1945: stipulations were added regarding the manufacture of fluoridated toothpaste, with the aim of removing fluoride from the country. But due to vested interests, this is proving a difficult task.

India was the first country in the world to develop protocols for diagnosing fluorosis at an early stage so that prevention of the disease was possible. Radiographs revealing skeletal fluorosis are of no use, because by the time skeletal fluorosis becomes apparent, it is too late to reverse the changes. Fluorosis has no treatment or cure. Prevention is the only solution, and for this, early diagnosis is essential.

For early detection, the two Indian protocols are (1) investigation of all gastrointestinal disturbances and (2) a sensitive blood test. At the same time, Indians are educated through radio, TV and the newspapers about the dangers of fluoride and how to avoid it.

The major problem is that, very often, skeletal fluorosis and non-skeletal fluorosis are misdiagnosed and treated wrongly, as clinicians do not fully understand the manifestations of fluoride poisoning. These are not described adequately in medical and dental textbooks.

Dental fluorosis is quite evident from the discoloration of the teeth. But Professor Susheela is convinced that dentists do not fully understand fluoride action on teeth, because they still promote fluoride among patients who already have dental fluorosis, despite the evidence of what is happening in India. She says: 'This truly reveals that no organisation or association can be taken for granted. Their intentions while promoting fluoride need to be questioned.'

India's ethical, up-to-date scientific research on fluoride toxicity contrasts strongly with the West's authoritarian fluoridation policy, based on low scientific standards and high political opinion.

The British situation

In its suggested answer to this question, the BFS states that the situation in Britain is quite different from that in India. In part, they are right. However, by saying that the Indian drinking water was different in that it 'was heavily contaminated with unsafe levels of natural chemicals including fluoride, arsenic, iron and salts', they are quite wrong. British (and Irish) drinking water in fluoridated areas is also contaminated with fluoride, arsenic, iron and salts.

As you can see from Figure 1, levels of fluoride in the drinking water in most of the areas that suffer endemic fluorosis in India – those marked with a square or a triangle – are *lower* than 3 ppm – a level the UK government tells us is safe.

The BFS is quite wrong in insisting that conditions such as skeletal fluorosis do not occur elsewhere in the fluoridated world. In Britain and Ireland, the number of cases of osteoporosis has been growing steadily over the past half-century. Osteoporosis now affects almost one in two post-menopausal women, and one in five of them will die as a direct result. It is also increasingly affecting men. One in six orthopaedic hospital beds were occupied by people with broken hips, at a cost to the NHS of £160 million per year by the mid-1980s.[2] Osteoporosis is caused by several factors. Many are related to advice given to the population by government: bran (cereal fibre) inhibits the absorption of calcium from diet,[3] low-fat diets also reduce calcium intake,[4] and fluoride displaces calcium and makes bones more brittle. Osteoporosis is regarded as merely 'a loss of calcium', without these other factors being taken into consideration; thus, the true extent of the role they play is obscured. In this way the BFS would have us believe that 'there is no evidence that skeletal fluorosis occurs'.

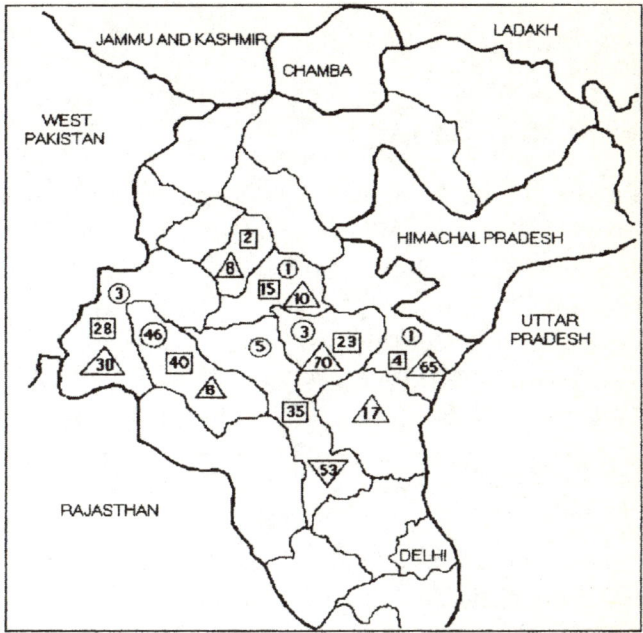

Figure 1. *Fluoride content of well water in endemic areas in India*

Source: WHO Fluorides and human health, Geneva: World Health Organisation, 1970

○ – *More than 3 ppm;* ❑ – *Between 1 and 3 ppm;* △ – *Less than 1ppm. Numerals indicate the number of specimens tested.*

Skeletal fluorosis

You would have to be naive in the extreme to believe that fluoride entering the body goes merely to the teeth. Fluorine has a particular affinity for calcium, wherever it is in the body. As calcium is most abundant in bones, fluorine moves rapidly to bones and other hard tissues, where most of it is retained while a fraction is excreted. But not all people are the same, and individual retention and excretion rates vary depending on three factors:

- Total fluoride intake

- Duration of exposure to fluoride

- Normal kidney function (adult males excrete more fluoride than females)

Fluoride's effects are cumulative: the mineral builds up over time. For this reason, any skeletal changes it causes progress through a number of stages, with the less serious changes occurring early in the natural course of the disease. Whatever may be the type of fluoride exposure, the clinical picture shows that chronic poisoning occurs in the following phased manner:[5]

1. **Preclinical phase:** Asymptomatic; slight radio-graphically detectable increases in bone mass

2. **Phase I (Musculoskeletal):** Sporadic pain; stiffness of joints; osteosclerosis of pelvis and spine

3. **Phase II (Degenerative and destructive):** Chronic joint pain; arthritic symptoms; slight calcification of ligaments; increased osteosclerosis/cancellous bones; with or without osteoporosis of long bones

4. **Phase III (Crippling fluorosis):** Limitation of joint movement; calcification of ligaments/neck, spinal column; crippling deformities of spine and major joints; muscle wasting; neurological defects/compression of spinal cord

Fluoride's effects depend not only on the total dosage and duration of exposure, but also on other factors, such as nutritional status, kidney function, and interactions with other trace elements. But what we really need to know is how much fluoride it takes before it begins to cause us harm.

You will remember that after the figures had been corrected, the amount needed to cause crippling fluorosis in a 100–229-pound person was reckoned to be 10–20 mg per day for ten to twenty years. Since fluorides accumulate in a linear fashion, the crippling dosage of 10 mg per day for ten years is the same as 5 mg per day for twenty years, and so on. If we extrapolate this to a normal lifetime drinking fluoridated water, this is the same as 2.5 mg per day for forty years. Using 2.5 mg as an example is not unreasonable: that is the amount of fluoride found in just 2.5 litres (less than 4.5 pints) of water!

It is also important to note that these figures are for *crippling fluorosis*, the last stage. It will take only four years at 10 mg per day, or sixteen years at 2.5 mg per day, before a 100-pound individual can expect to experience Phase I – musculoskeletal fluorosis – with chronic joint pain and arthritic symptoms, with or without osteoporosis.

Based on the figures in the NAS/NRC's 1993 report, *Health Effects of Ingested Fluoride*, and on those published by Hodge in 1979, Table 1 shows the minimum daily fluoride intake associated with the development of crippling skeletal fluorosis, according to body weight and years of exposure.

The American chemist Bette Hileman was scathing of the lack of studies into skeletal fluorosis carried out in her own country, saying:

> Although skeletal fluorosis has been studied intensely in other countries for more than 40 years, virtually no research has been done in the US to determine how many people are afflicted with the earlier stages of the disease, particularly the preclinical stages. Because some of the clinical symptoms mimic arthritis, the first two clinical phases of skeletal fluorosis could be easily misdiagnosed. Skeletal fluorosis is not even discussed in most medical texts under the effects of fluoride; indeed, a number of texts say the condition is almost

nonexistent in the US. Even if a doctor is aware of the disease, the early stages are difficult to diagnose.[6]

Body weight (lb)	Minimum mg/day for 11 years	Minimum mg/day for 44 years
229	20.77	5.19
220	19.96	4.99
210	19.05	4.76
200	18.14	4.54
190	17.24	4.31
180	16.32	4.08
170	15.42	3.86
160	14.52	3.63
150	13.6	3.4
140	12.7	3.18
130	11.79	2.95
120	10.89	2.72
110	9.98	2.49
100	9.07	2.27

Note: Intake figures by body weight for 44 years are shown here for purposes of comparison only.

Source: *Health effects of ingested fluoride.* Subcommittee on Health Effects of Ingested Fluoride, Committee on Toxicology, Board on Environmental Studies and Toxicology, Commission on Life Sciences, US National Research Council, August 1993.

Table 1. Minimum daily fluoride intake associated with Phase III skeletal fluorosis

Bone changes observed in human skeletal fluorosis are structural and functional, with a combination of osteosclerosis, osteomalacia, osteoporosis, and exostosis formation, as well as secondary hyperparathyroidism in a proportion of patients.

Fluoride weakens bones

About 10 per cent of bone tissue is broken down and replaced each year. At this stage, any ingested fluoride is incorporated in the new bone structure. Because of fluoride's affinity for calcium, in 1961 Dr C. Rich originated a treatment for osteoporosis, administering large doses of fluoride in the belief that the fluoride would assist the formation of new bone substance, strengthening it and preventing fracture. At first it looked as if the scheme might be successful: as expected, the bones of women who took the fluoride supplements looked considerably denser on X-rays and bone scans. But although the bones looked denser, they were weaker. Women treated with fluoride supplements had significantly more fractures. Five years after he began, Rich also warned that there were other side effects: gastric pain, calcification of the arteries, osteoarthritis and visual disturbances.[7] The treatment was abandoned.

But the weakening of bones doesn't happen only with supplements. All fluoride weakens bones. For this reason, it can be predicted that as people ingest more fluoride in water or food, so the rate of osteoporotic fractures will increase. And so it proves to be. Numbers of hip fractures have risen dramatically among both women and men since water fluoridation began.

In 1978 scientists at Yale University reported that fluoride in strengths as little as the 'optimal' 1 ppm decreased bone strength and elasticity.[8] Workers at the Roswell Park Memorial Institute also showed that fluoride accelerated the process of osteoporosis.[9] In 1992, a study of elderly patients in Utah found 'a small but significant increase in the risk of hip fracture in both men and women exposed to artificial fluoridation at 1 part per million'.[10] The relative risk of hip fracture in the higher-fluoride group, compared with the lower-fluoride group, was 27 per cent greater for women and 41 per cent greater for men. Figure 2 shows the data for men from this study. Dr John R. Lee concluded from this study that '[f]luoride is toxic to bones and increases risk of fracture at all levels of exposure including fluoridation at 1 ppm. Regardless of any other consideration, this is reason enough to discontinue fluoridation immediately.'[11]

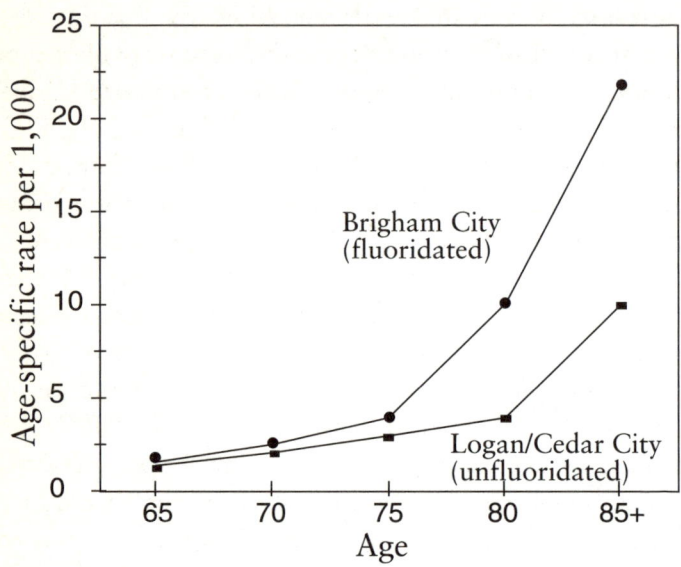

Source: Danielson et al. *J Am Med Assoc* 1992; 268: 746–8.

Figure 2. Hip fractures, rate per 1,000, men

The total quantity of fluoride ingested is the single most important factor in determining the clinical course of skeletal fluorosis; the severity of symptoms correlates directly with the level and duration of exposure.[12] The WHO recognised this thirty years ago, which is why the WHO called for *all* sources of fluoride to be considered before decisions to fluoridate are taken. In 1970 the WHO said:

> At higher levels of ingestion – from 2 to 8 mg daily, skeletal fluorosis may arise . . . Whereas dental fluorosis

is easily recognized, the skeletal involvement is not clinically obvious until the advanced stage of crippling fluorosis . . . early cases may be misdiagnosed as rheumatoid or osteoarthritis.[13]

With fluoride in food (whether due to pesticides or to the use of fluoridated water in food processing), water, toothpaste, air, and so on, 2–8 mg daily is easily within people's intakes even if they live in areas that do not have fluoridated drinking water.

In recent years, four additional studies have demonstrated an increased incidence of hip fractures among elderly people living in fluoridated areas. Jacobsen (USA), Cooper (UK) and Colquhoun (New Zealand) all state that increased fracture of the hip has occurred since the advent of fluoridation.[14] Colquhoun said: 'I find it astonishing therefore that, at a time when women's hip fractures in New Zealand are reaching epidemic proportions, health boards are still claiming that fluoridated water is perfectly safe.' Dr C. Danielson and colleagues conclude: 'Fluoridation of water supplies was initiated prior to long-term studies of its effects on bone density. Recent studies suggest that fluoride accumulates with age and may reach toxic bone levels in a person's lifetime (at a water content of 0.97 ppm).'[15]

According to Dr Lee there have been 'seven studies showing a positive correlation of fluoridation with increased hip fracture incidence and not one acceptable study showing the contrary'.[16]

Conclusion

Skeletal fluorosis has been studied extensively in India and other countries for more than forty years, whereas almost no research has been done in the USA, Britain, Ireland or other artificially fluoridating countries. Don't be misled by the BFS statement that 'in temperate climates, such as the UK, USA and Canada, there is no evidence that skeletal fluorosis occurs'. Absence of evidence is not the same as evidence of absence. Many symptoms of skeletal fluorosis – osteoporosis, spondylosis, and other bone conditions – are there to be found. Are they caused by fluoride? I suspect they are, as levels of fluoride intake in Britain and Ireland are not so very different from those in India, where skeletal fluorosis is documented. But we will never know for sure until the situation is taken seriously.

References

1. Susheela AK. Letter to Rotary International, Oakmont, PA, 24 February 1996.
2. Editorial. Why so many fractured hips? *Lancet* 1989; i: 57.
3. Suri YP. The bran wagon. *Lancet* 1987; ii: 42–3.
4. Reynolds JJ. *Boneturnover, vitamin D and plasma calcium homeostasis*. In Talmage RV, Owen M, Parsons JA (eds) *Calcium Regulating Hormones*. Excerpta Medica, Amsterdam, 1975.
5. Mertz W, ed. *Trace elements in human and animal nutrition*, 5th edn. US Department of Agriculture, Agricultural Research Service, Beltsville Human Nutrition Research Center, Beltsville, MD, 1987: 368.
6. Hileman B. *Fluoridation of water*. Special report. *Chem Eng News* 1 August 1988: 35–6.
7. Waldbott GL, in collaboration with Burgstahler A, McKinney HL. *Fluoridation: The great dilemma*. Lawrence, KS: Coronado Press, 1978: 81–4.
8. Albright JA. The effect of fluoride on the mechanical properties of bone. *Trans Ann Meet Orthopedics Res Soc* 1978; 240 (15): 1630–1.
9. Robin JC, Schepart B, Calkins H et al. Studies on osteoporosis III. Effect of estrogens and fluoride. *J Med* 1980; 11 (1): 1–14.

10. Danielson C, Lyon JL, Egger M, Goodenough GK. Hip fractures and fluoridation in Utah's elderly population. *J Am Med Assoc* 1992; 268: 746–8.

11. Lee JR. Fluoridation and osteoporosis: The facts. *Health Freedom News* January 1994: 26.

12. *Review of fluoride: Benefits and risks.* US Department of Health and Human Services, February 1991: 45.

13. WHO. *Fluorides and human health.* Geneva: World Health Organization, 1970: 239.

14. Jacobsen, S, Goldberg J et al. Regional variation in the incidence of hip fracture: US white women aged 65 years and older. *J Am Med Assoc* 1990; 264: 500–2. Cooper C, Whickham C et al. Water fluoride concentration and fracture of the proximal femur. *J Epidemioc Community Health* 1990; 44: 17–19, and Water fluoridation and hip fracture. *J Am Med Assoc* 1991; 266: 513–4. Colquhoun J. Water fluoride and fractures. *NZ med J* 1991; 104: 343.

15. Danielson C, Lyon JL, Egger M, Goodenough GK. Hip fractures and fluoridation in Utah's elderly population. *J Am Med Assoc* 1992; 268: 746–8.

16. Lee JR. Fluoridation and hip fracture according to the National Research Council report: 'Health effects of ingested fluoride'. *Fluoride* 1993; 26: 274–7.

29. The Public and Fluoride

Does the public want fluoridation?

BFS suggested answer

Yes. National opinion surveys conducted by NOP and Gallup consistently show that around 70% of the public believe that fluoride should be added to water supplies to prevent tooth decay.

In addition, statutory local consultations conducted by over 60 health authorities have demonstrated a high level of public support.

BFS suggested answer refuted

We have exhausted every democratic avenue and it is out of frustration that we are knocking on Tony Worthington's door. More than half of the adult population concerned has asked for fluoridation to stop. They are over 18 and taxpayers and they don't want fluoridation – even if it were good for them.
Walter Graham

In November 1996, John Hunt, chief executive of the British Dental Association, reported:

> A majority of MPs, the general public, and all the major public health organisations support water fluoridation as a safe and effective way of defeating tooth decay. At present only 10% of the population receive fluoridated water: a target of 25% by the end of the century must be set so that people all over the country are able to benefit from improved dental health.[1]

British Dental Association poll of members of parliament

Tom Braithwaite, the Liberal Democrat spokesman on water, stated at the British Fluoridation Society's meeting in Westminster in November 1997 that the Liberal Democrats were in favour of fluoridation (despite the fact that no party has a policy on fluoridation) and that 'as 70 per cent of all MPs were in favour, legislation would succeed'. John Hunt seemed to confirm this when he gave figures for the three major parties. Putting to MPs the question: 'Do you believe that fluoride should be added to water if it can reduce tooth decay?', he reported the following answers:

- Of 256 Labour MPs who answered, 77 per cent were in favour of fluoridation.

- Of 113 Conservative MPs who answered, 62 per cent were in favour of fluoridation.

- Of 34 Liberal Democrat MPs who answered, 65 per cent were in favour of fluoridation.

This is the origin of the 70 per cent figure. But this survey of MPs was misleading: the 70 per cent figure related only to those MPs who answered the question – and that was only about half of the total who had been asked. In other words, it was 70 per cent of 50 per cent, which is in reality only 35 per cent known to be in favour of fluoridation.

The Green Party, on the other hand, is 100 per cent opposed to it, calling for the repeal of all existing legislation permitting water fluoridation.

Polls of the public by BFS

The 70 per cent figure is also remarkably consistent when public polls are conducted by the BFS. But as any trained interviewer or pollster knows, the answer to any question can be influenced by the way the question is worded. For example, early in 2000, in a demonstration of people's willingness to sign petitions, passers-by in New York were asked to sign a petition calling for an end to women's suffrage. 'Suffrage', of course, has nothing to do with suffering; suffrage is the right to vote. Yet hundreds of people, including women, signed the petition.

The question the BFS asks is: 'Do you believe that fluoride should be added to water if it can reduce tooth decay?' The addition of the words 'if it can reduce tooth decay' ensures that those questioned will be more likely to give an affirmative answer. Such a question would never be allowed in a court of law. Most people are not very knowledgeable about the fluoridation issue because of the secrecy surrounding it. If the question were alternatively worded – 'Do you think that people should be medicated without their consent?' – what would the answer be?

Contrast the polls by pro-fluoridationists with a survey carried out in Britain in 1993 by the Office of Population Censuses and Surveys,[2] which asked people how one attains good dental hygiene. The majority mentioned things like brushing teeth, visiting the dentist, and limiting sugar in the diet. Less than 5 per cent mentioned fluoride as a key factor.

A survey published in the *British Dental Journal* in May 2000, asking whether people wanted to be involved in the decision-making process when water fluoridation was mooted for their area, demonstrated the public's lack of knowledge.[3] You might expect that people who value their health, and who are being prescribed a drug whose sole purpose is to change their bodies' chemical composition, would want to be involved in the decision about whether or not they take that drug. Yet the study found that the public did not want to be involved in the decision-making process. The study concluded that they 'do not see themselves as being the appropriate implementation arbiters'. In this, they show far more sense than the dentists asking the questions.

Other polls of the public in Britain

The British Dental Association and the British Fluoridation Society are not the only ones to conduct polls about fluoridation. Local councils have done it, as have newspapers and TV. These polls have come up with quite different findings: not 70 per cent in favour of fluoridation, but as many as 98 per cent against it.

The only British referendum

The level of fluoride occurring naturally in the drinking water of the residents of Bolton, Lancashire, was 0.1–0.2 ppm in 1965. In that year the Bolton Borough Council agreed that fluoride should be added to bring the total up to 1.0 ppm. In 1968 the Waterworks Committee made preparations to add fluoride to two reservoirs that supplied Bolton's drinking water. But because an 'extraordinary controversy' had been aroused by the proposal, Bolton's Health Committee met on 24 July 1968 to discuss 'fluoridation of the water supplies'. When the full council met on 7 August 1968, Bolton Borough Council decided to defer fluoridation for the time being and ordered a referendum to be held on the question of fluoridation. The results, announced to the Health Committee on 23 October 1968, were:[4]

For fluoridation	23,596 (27 per cent)
Against fluoridation	63,290 (73 per cent)

This referendum is important as the only referendum ever carried out in Britain to assess the wishes of the population on the matter of fluoridation. It was also important for another reason: the 82 per cent turnout was one of the highest ever seen in the town for any purpose, even higher than most turnouts for a general election. This demonstrated the strength of feeling about, and overwhelming distrust of, fluoridation.

In 1998, after the British government published its Green Paper, *Our Healthier Nation*, there was again widespread concern among the people of Bolton. As a consequence, the *Bolton Evening News* conducted a telephone poll of its readers. This time, a staggering 95 per cent of callers were against fluoride.[5]

North-west England

Calderdale was to be fluoridated in the 1970s. In 1978, Dennis Edmondson alone collected 23,000 signatures on a petition against fluoridation in that town. As a result, Calderdale Town Council obtained an injunction preventing the addition of fluoride. Since then, almost every local council in the north-west has voted against fluoridation. Feeling was so strong that, on an initiative of Barrow-in-Furness Town Council, a consortium of sixteen councils, to be called North West Councils Against Fluoridation (NWCAF), was set up to fight fluoridation. Today, twenty-eight of the thirty-one city and district councils north of High Peak in Derbyshire are members of NWCAF. The north-western health authorities wanted fluoridation, but North West Water turned down their requests repeatedly for four years. In June 1992 the company told the health authorities that the 'councils' views were the opinion of the majority of their customers'. The very next day, a dentist in a radio interview about this decision accused NWCAF of killing children!

Manchester

Manchester, Salford and Trafford councils are not members of NWCAF. In a *Manchester Evening News* telephone poll in November 1998, 92 per cent voted against fluoridation.[6]

Southampton and Hampshire

A poll conducted in Southampton and south Hampshire in 1997 found 90 per cent of people were against fluoridation.[7]

Leicester

Leicestershire Health Authority voted to add fluoride to drinking water in 1989. There was an uproar when the then chairman, George Farnham, used his casting vote to force through the decision – as he sat there with a bottle of mineral water in front of him.

The *Leicester Mercury* conducted the first telephone poll in its history on this issue – and received 66,000 calls. 'Of all the phone polls we have had over the years, it was by far and away the biggest we have ever had.' The decision of the Health Authority was overturned when 94 per cent of callers opposed fluoridation.[8]

Glasgow

The result of an 'extensive' *Glasgow Evening Times* poll in August 2000 was a 98 per cent vote against fluoridation. This beat a similar 'massive' poll by the *Glasgow Evening Times* in October 1999, in which 97 per cent were against fluoridation. Liz Vaughan, spokesperson for North West Councils and Northern Ireland Councils Against Fluoridation, said:

> This is another indicator to government that the public rejects their claims of safety. Furthermore, the people view such a practice – which is mass medication without consent – as grossly unethical. It seems that the BDA and the British Fluoridation Society do not understand the word 'NO', and their determination to fluoridate the drinking water is now being widely seen as public harassment.

Northern Ireland

Twenty-five of the twenty-six elected councils across Northern Ireland rejected fluoridation after the last public consultation in Northern Ireland ended on 12 April 1996. They were supported by the four Health and Social Services Councils, MPs, the Ulster Farmers' Union, the Northern Ireland Agricultural Producers' Association, environment groups, anglers, and the people. But despite this emphatic No to fluoridation in Northern Ireland, it is still pressed on people there.

In 1998, following two years of discontent with an officialdom that refused to answer questions or give adequate responses, the patience of the people of two small but significant towns, Holywood and Tandragee, finally ran out, and they picketed the government buildings at Stormont. 'We have exhausted every democratic avenue and it is out of frustration that we are knocking on Tony Worthington's door,' said Walter Graham. 'More than half of the adult population concerned has asked for fluoridation to stop. They are over 18 and taxpayers and they don't want fluoridation – even if it were good for them.'

A subsequent statement released by the Department of Health said that fluoridation continued to be part of the dental health promotion policy. What kind of Minister for Health ignores such strong representations in a supposedly free and democratic country?

The Channel Islands

Residents in Jersey and Guernsey asked the National Pure Water Association for urgent help after the islands' health departments began proclaiming the benefits of artificial fluoridation. They were not just worried about their own health. Channel Islanders were also worried that tourists from unfluoridated France and Germany might be reluctant to visit the Channel Islands if the health departments went ahead with their plans.

Teletext poll

In 1999, Channel 4's Teletext conducted a telephone poll. More than 700 people called in. That might not seem a lot, but a spokesman for Teletext said that, for them, it was a huge response showing the strength of feeling there was on the issue. In this poll, 97 per cent were against fluoridation.

Ireland

Even though fluoridation is a legal requirement in Ireland, the people don't want it. Dublin City Council adopted this motion on 1 March 1999:

> That this City Council calls on the Manager to remove fluoride from the drinking water supply in light of scientific evidence that the health risks associated with fluoride may well outweigh any benefit from reduction in dental caries. Most European countries do not use fluoride in their water supplies and have at least as good a record on oral hygiene as Ireland and requests the Taoiseach to set up an expert technical group to review the medical, dental and environmental effects of fluoridation of water.

Donegal County Council passed the following motion on 13 December 1999: 'That Donegal County Council would suspend the fluoridation of water pending the outcome of an investigation by the Oireachtas Committee on Health and Children on the effects of fluoridation in water'.

Sligo County Council, on 6 March 2000, unanimously adopted the motion: 'That Sligo County Council calls upon the Government and Minister for Health to amend the Health

(Fluoridation of Water Supplies) Act 1960, so as to allow local authorities to make the final decision on whether drinking water should be fluoridated'.

Clare County Council, on 28 November 2000, passed the following motion: 'This council seeks through Longford County Council and the Midland Health Board to have the Health (Fluoridation of Water Supplies) Act 1960, which requires the mandatory fluoridation of water, revoked by the Minister of Health and Children in the National Interest.'

Leitrim County Council passed the following motion unanimously on 4 December 2000: 'That this council calls on the Minister of Health to immediately amend the Act which makes the fluoridation of water mandatory and that the minister allows the county councils to make their own decision in the matter'.

But such motions were overruled by the Irish Department of Health.[9]

Conclusion

The results of polls not commissioned by the BFS totally contradict claims that the public supports fluoridation. With all polls, one needs to keep in mind that the results of a poll depend very much upon the way a question is asked.

People are learning that there are two sides to the fluoride debate. According to a 1990 letter from the Florida Department of Health and Rehabilitative Services, '[T]he statistics are that three out of four fluoridation referenda fail.' The letter highlighted this point by suggesting that communities wishing to fluoridate should 'avoid a referendum'.[10]

References

1. Dentists urge public to ignore unscientific claims of anti-fluoride groups. British Dental Association news release, WWW-PR22. 13 November 1996.
2. O'Brien M. *Children's dental health in the United Kingdom.* Social Survey Division, Office of Population, Census and Surveys (OPCS), 1993.
3. Lowry RJ, Thompson B, Lennon MA. How much do the general public want to be involved in decisions on implementing water fluoridation? *Br Dent J* 2000; 188: 500–2.
4. *Fluoridation.* Annual Report of the Medical Officer of Health, County Borough of Bolton, UK, 31 December 1968: 168.
5. Battle plan: Bolton to host summit talks on compulsory fluoridation. *Bolton Evening News*, 20–21 February 1999.
6. *Manchester Evening News*, 2 November 1998 and 4 November 1998.
7. Outrage over water probe. *Southern Daily Echo* (United Kingdom), 21 October 1997.
8. Preparing to sink their teeth into new battle. *Leicester Mercury*, 17 July 2000.
9. Fluoride in our water: are we brushing with danger? Special report. *Irish Independent*, 29 March 2000.
10. http://www.fluoridealert.org/low-profile.htm. Accessed 26 August 2000.

30. Legislating for Fluoride

> ## Why do we need a campaign for water fluoridation?
>
> **BFS suggested answer**
> Only around 10% of the UK population currently receives fluoridated water mainly in the West Midlands and the North East of England. However, over 60 health authorities are being prevented from implementing water fluoridation policies because current legislation is flawed.
>
> **BFS suggested answer refuted**
> *The passion to regulate the lives of others is deep-seated in many individuals. When this is based on political expediency, it is bad, and when it is inspired by an idealism which wishes to inflict benefit on others, it can be dangerous.*
> Sir Arthur Amies

Despite pressure from the British Fluoridation Society, the British Dental Association, and other health authorities for over fifty years, only about 9 per cent of the population of England and Wales drinks fluoridated water. The reason given by the BFS for this is that 'legislation is flawed'. What they mean by this is in the wording of the Water (Fluoridation) Act 1985, which states:

> 1.B(1) Where a health authority have applied in writing to a statutory water undertaker for the water supplied within an area specified in the application to be fluoridated, that undertaker may, while the application remains in force, increase the fluoride content of the water supplied by them within that area.

The bone of contention in this subsection, as far as the fluoride lobbyists are concerned, is the inclusion of the word 'may'. This gives the water companies the option of refusing to comply with a health authority's request, thus giving the water company the final say on whether to add fluoride to the water.

Section 4 of the Act requires health authorities wishing to add fluoride to drinking water to publish details of the proposal in local newspapers and give notice of it to every local authority whose area falls wholly or partly within the area affected by the fluoridation proposal, at least three months before its implementation. This section also requires the health authority to consult each of the local authorities affected by the proposal and take note of their wishes. Before the proposal to fluoridate goes ahead, the health authority is required to consider any representations that have been made to it and any consultations that have taken place with interested parties.

But the health authority is not bound by these representations and consultations – and it shows. Over the years, even where local authorities and people in the community have told the health authority that they do not want fluoride, health authorities have invariably overridden these objections and requested water companies to put fluoride in the drinking water anyway.

The evidence given in the previous chapter demonstrates that people do not want fluoride. The water companies know this, and mindful that they will carry the can if anyone is harmed by fluoride, no water company has added fluoride to its drinking water since the 1985 Act, even though some sixty requests for fluoridation have been made by health authorities to water companies since the Act became law.

Dentists and health authorities see these failures to fluoridate as a conspiracy by the water companies to thwart their efforts to improve the dental health of the nation. They refuse to accept that people do not want fluoride.

This so-called 'flaw' has prompted the pro-fluoride lobby to make a concerted effort to get the law changed in order to *compel* water companies to add fluoride.

The plot thickens

But there is a second subtle twist to the plot. At present, all local councillors at district, town and county level discuss, debate and vote on all matters within their jurisdiction. Meetings, both of committees and the full council, are open to the public and press. The British government proposes to change this so that decisions will be taken by a 'Cabinet' rather than by the whole council. The government also proposes to shift decision-making on fluoridation away from health authorities and give it to local councils. This means that a small caucus of councillors within the ruling political group, which is likely to dominate political activity in the council, will decide whether their district or town shall be fluoridated.

Local councillors are chosen and elected by their people; area health authorities, on the other hand, are unelected officials. By shifting the responsibility for fluoridation from health authorities to local councils, the British government is giving the impression that it is making the process more democratic. But the proposed shift from open government to Cabinet-style government, with decisions being taken in camera, thus excluding the public and the press, makes the process even more suspect that it is at present.

Local government insurance

The new human rights legislation in the UK came into force on 2 October 2000. With the introduction of that legislation, all authorities, whether local or state, government or other public or private bodies, that are involved in the fluoridation process will become liable not only for the infringement of those rights but also for compensation for any resulting adverse effects, both in the future and in the past.

Eighty per cent of local government authorities and a huge number of other public-sector organisations, including NHS Trusts, are insured with Zurich Municipal. According to Rachel Coventry, Zurich's local government marketing controller:

> The incorporation of the European Convention on Human Rights into domestic law could land organisations that fail to prepare in court, but many of the dangers can be foreseen. Local authorities can help to protect themselves by conducting audits to assess the compliance with the new requirements. Those that don't could find themselves paying the price.[1]

The implications of the legislation are clear: it appears that government and its lower echelons have much to learn about their responsibilities to the public.

Conclusion

The people of Britain, like people in most other countries, don't want fluoride added to their drinking water. It seems to me that the reason that this campaign is thought necessary by the BFS is that only by compulsion can people be forced to take this toxic substance against their wishes. As Sir Arthur Amies said, it's a dangerous business – as local councils deciding on fluoridation would do well to consider.

References

1. Councils given six-month Human Rights Act warning. 29 March 2000. http://www.zurichmunicipal.com/localauthorities/press/med20000329_6_month_warning. htm. Accessed 2 May 2000.

31. Fluoride Not an Essential Nutrient

Do we need to fluoridate all water supplies?

BFS suggested answer

No. The British Dental Association recommends that coverage should be extended to reach 25% of the population where tooth decay rates are unacceptably high. These areas include: the West of Scotland, the North West and parts of the North East of England, parts of Yorkshire, parts of Wales, and Inner London.

BFS suggested answer refuted

Fluoride does not need to be swallowed to be effective. It is not an essential nutrient. Nor should it be considered a desirable 'supplement' for children living in non-fluoridated areas . . . Even if there were a systemic benefit from ingestion of fluoride, it would be minuscule and clinically irrelevant. The notion that systemic fluorides are needed in non-fluoridated areas is an outdated one that should be abandoned altogether.
Hardy Limeback, associate professor and head of preventive dentistry, University of Toronto

A major argument that fluoridationists put forward in favour of fluoridation is that fluoride is essential for the correct formation of dental enamel. In other words, fluorine is an element that the body needs to develop healthily: an essential nutrient, in the same way as other minerals and vitamins.

FDA position on 'nutrient' fluoride

New rules for recommended daily allowances (RDAs) for

nutrients were proposed by the US Food and Drugs Administration (FDA) in the early 1970s. In January 1973 the FDA published a list of several nutrients that were termed essential but for which no RDAs had been established. Fluorine was included in this list.[1] Later that year, fluoride was officially classified as essential by the FDA.[2] Yet, strangely, despite this classification of 'essential' given to fluoride, dietary supplements containing fluoride were, and still are, available only on prescription.

The following year, as a result of court action challenging some of the FDA's policies and regulations, the FDA was ordered to integrate into the Code of Federal Regulations (CFR) those nutrients, including fluoride, that were classified as essential but that did not have RDAs. These nutrients would then be available for food additives or dietary supplements.[3]

In 1975, the FDA explicitly designated fluoride as '*not* generally recognized as safe'.[4] Any vitamin or mineral that is not generally recognised as safe falls into the 'food additive' category under the Federal Food, Drug and Cosmetics Act 1945. And so, fluoride was placed in this category. Unlike many other substances, which become food additives only if they exceed a certain level, fluoride is a food additive at any level.

The FDA permits no fluoride whatsoever to be added to food or over-the-counter dietary supplements – it is not designated as safe at any level. Despite this, the Department of Health, Education and Welfare exempted fluoridated water supplies from this FDA ban.[5] It also exempted the addition of such fluoridated water in the processing of food.[6]

By 1976 fluoride's classification as essential was downgraded to 'probably essential', for which no RDA was established.[7] And three years later, the FDA deleted the paragraphs of the *Federal Register* that had classified fluorine as essential or probably essential.[8] From March 1979, fluoride ceased to be either an essential or a probably essential nutrient in the USA.

In 1991 the US public health service reported: 'Although fluoride compounds occur naturally, both in the environment and in most constituents of the body, there is no conclusive evidence that fluorine or any of the fluoride compounds are essential for human homeostasis or growth.'[9]

The 'belief' by fluoride proponents that our bodies need fluoride is just that – a belief. It's not based on scientific research.

Dietary Reference Values for Food Energy and Nutrients for the United Kingdom

The latest edition of this book was published by the UK Department of Health in 1997.[10] That was the year in which the Department of Health increased its funding of the British Fluoridation Society from £74,000 to £117,000 a year.

The chapter on fluoride is the only one that has a heading announcing: 'This chapter and the safe intake levels have been revised to take account of some inconsistencies within the previous chapter.' One of the 'inconsistencies' was a reference in the previous edition to the fact that '[w]here the water supply naturally contains 1 mg/kg (1 ppm), early radiographic evidence of skeletal fluorosis has been reported in adult populations'. It was removed.

The Panel on the Dietary Reference Values quotes the British Dental Association's 1981 recommendation that fluoride supplements were necessary in unfluoridated areas. It missed the *British Dental Journal*'s explicit statement of 11 January 1997: 'Fluoride supplements are no longer generally seen as a public health measure where water fluoridation has not been introduced.'

The Panel omitted another 'inconsistent' scientific reference in the previous edition: 'In the USA infants and children who received fluoride supplements of 0.5 mg/day until 3 years of age and 1.0 mg/day thereafter had a 63%

incidence of dental fluorosis by the age of 12 years.' These supplement dosages are essentially the same as those recommended by the British Dental Association in 1981.

Nowhere does the Panel refer to the fact that 50 per cent of all fluoride ingested will accumulate in the skeleton and that this continues throughout life into old age. The Panel has ducked the consideration of any aspect of this accumulation in bone in British fluoridated areas by quoting American research in Texas in 1950 and the results of an Australian enquiry in 1980.[11]

As in previous editions, the publication had to admit: 'No essential function for fluoride has been proven in humans.' It states: 'As there does not appear to be a physiological requirement for fluoride the Panel set no Reference Nutritional Intake.' But that didn't stop the Panel endorsing water fluoridation.

This latest publication includes a chapter on sugars. The Panel accepts the conclusions of COMA's 1989 report, which stated that 'sugars were a major cause of dental caries in the UK and that their consumption by the population should be decreased'.[12]

Despite the fact that medical experts in the UK Department of Health are obviously aware of the pre-eminent role of sugar in causing dental decay, the Welsh and English Green Papers, which purport to consider all aspects of health, make no mention of sugar at all, preferring instead to concentrate solely on fluoridation as the ideal remedy for tooth decay.

Conclusion

Dentists invariably misguide the public by designating dental caries as a fluoride deficiency disorder. But this is a gross scientific error. We know from Chapter 1 that you can have perfectly good teeth without fluoride. Our bodies have no need of it.

There can be no such thing as a fluoride deficiency, as fluorine is such a ubiquitous element. Fluoride is not a nutrient: it is used only as a medication, with the supposed therapeutic effects of strengthening the tooth enamel and killing off the oral bacteria that cause tooth decay.

There are more sensible ways of giving fluoride to those who want it. If we choose to ignore the risks of fluoride and set as our goal the adequate provision of fluoride for children's teeth, the most sensible way to reach that goal is to use toothpaste and the numerous fluoride-containing dental products.

So the truthful answer to this question is: No. Britain doesn't need to fluoridate *any* water supplies.

References

1. Vol 38, *Fed Reg* 2149 (19 January 1973).
2. Vol 38, *Fed Reg* 20717 (2 August 1973).
3. *National Nutritional Foods Association (NNFA)* v. FDA, 504 *Federal Reporter* 2d, p. 786; Court of Appeals, Second Circuit, decided 15 August 1974.
4. Vol 40, *Fed Reg* 23248 (28 May 1975).
5. CFR, Title 21, 1979, Par. 170.45: 'Fluorine-containing compounds'.
6. CFR, Title 21, 1979, Par. 250.203: 'Status of fluoridated water and food prepared with fluoridated water'.
7. Vol 41, *Fed Reg* 46175 (19 October 1976).
8. Vol 44, *Fed Reg* 16006 (16 March 1979).
9. *Review of fluoride: Benefits and risks.* US Department of Health and Human Services, 1991.
10. UK Department of Health. *Report on health and social subjects. 41: Dietary reference values for food energy and nutrients for the United Kingdom.* 8th impression. London: HMSO, 1997.

11. *Victoria Committee report of fluoridation of Victorian water supplies.* Melbourne: FD Atkinson, Government printer, 1980: 278.
12. UK Department of Health. *Report on health and social subjects.* 37: *Dietary sugars and human disease.* London: HMSO, 1989.

32. Fluoride and Controversy

Why is fluoridation so controversial?

BFS suggested answer
There is no scientific controversy over fluoridation. A small number of determined, vocal, but misguided campaigners refuse to accept the incontrovertible facts that fluoridation is safe and effective. In the words of the US Consumer's Union, 'the survival of this fake controversy represents one of the major triumphs of quackery over science in our generation.'

National opinion surveys conducted by NOP and Gallup consistently show that around 70% of the public believe that fluoride should be added to water supplies to prevent tooth decay.

BFS suggested answer refuted
The point is that this is a legitimate scientific controversy. Proponents of fluoridation insist that there are no grounds for controversy at all, and with that, I totally disagree.
Dr Edward Groth III

The long-running nature of the controversy about fluoridation and the strength of feeling on both sides of the divide is caused by the unwillingness of those in favour of fluoride even to consider that there might be adverse effects in humans – despite the fact that there is no dispute that fluoride can and does harm plants, birds, fish, insects and mammals.

The fluoridation controversy is symptomatic of a deep-seated pathology in present-day science. The magnitude of that malady motivated the US Academy of Sciences to convene a Panel on Scientific Responsibility and the Conduct of Research.[1] The Panel's investigation, which cost $888,000, precluded consideration of certain kinds of scientific misconduct that apply specifically to fluoridation. This misconduct occurs, according to Joel Griffiths, 'when new scientific evidence threatens fluoride's protected pollutant status. The government immediately appoints a commission, typically composed of several veteran fluoride defenders and no opponents. Usually, these commissions dismiss the new evidence and reaffirm the status quo. When one didn't in 1983, the government simply altered the findings.'[2]

The controversy about fluoridation is inevitable because fluoridation was, in a real sense, conceived in sin. Fluoride is one of industry's most devastating pollutants. Yet the US government not only dismissed the danger and left industry free to pollute, it promoted the addition of that fluoride to drinking water. The same is happening in Britain, the Republic of Ireland and other countries. Since fluoridation was first sanctioned over half a century ago, millions of tons of fluoride have been pumped into the environment via the water supply. Don't forget that these exact same chemicals, if allowed to escape into the atmosphere, are 'hazardous air pollutants'.

Blatant disregard for people's health

Before fluoride was considered as an anti-caries treatment, the American Dental Association recognised that it was toxic, that it caused fluorosis, that fluorosis was undesirable, and that fluoride should therefore be removed from drinking water. Now, as the result of sustained pressure from industry, fluorosis is a condition to be desired – so long as it is not too noticeable.

But the toxicity has not gone away. According to Dr Hobart T. Feldman, of the American Board of Allergy and Immunology:

> Fluoride is capable of producing any number of symptoms . . . [they] include drowsiness, profound desire

to sleep, dizziness, nasal congestion, sneezing, runny nose, sore throat, coughing, wheezing (asthma), chest pain, hives, and various intestinal symptoms. One reason for the lack of information in current medical literature, is the fact that these symptoms have been observed by private practising physicians, who accept such reactions as being related to specific chemical compounds, but are too busy in their practices to attempt to formulate a comprehensive investigative report which would satisfy the editorial positions of many of the journals and medical newspapers. Nevertheless, I can assure you that any of the above reactions can and do occur in significant numbers of people. Case reports are rarely accepted in the medical literature. Therefore, most of the information concerning specific reactions to fluoride, as seen in private practice, never reach publication.[3]

This secrecy has undermined any trust that could once have been placed in the word of a dentist. Fluoridation of water is only one source of fluoride in our environment. The amount that finds its way into our bodies from drinking fluoridated water is no longer even the major portion. In 1993, the Committee on Toxicology of the US National Research Council stated:

The most effective approach to stabilizing the prevalence and severity of dental fluorosis, without jeopardizing the benefits to oral health, is likely to come from more judicious control of fluoride in foods, processed beverages, and dental products, rather than a reduction in the recommended concentrations of fluoride in drinking water. But applying such a policy would be formidable; reduction of fluoride concentrations in drinking water would be easier to administer, monitor, and evaluate.[4]

Whichever way you look at it, there is now so much fluoride

around that water fluoridation is unnecessary, and would still be unnecessary even if it worked.

Conclusion

Pro-fluoridationists don't want water fluoridation debated, and, of course, after more than half a century of fluoridating water, there should by now be no *reason* for a debate. There is no debate within the scientific community that fluorides are toxic. Under the circumstances, safety tests should have been done decades ago and the whole business settled, *before* the first cities were fluoridated. But even now, those safety tests have yet to be done.

Those who maintain that fluoride is safe have only their faith to back their belief; there are no data to back their claims. Those who maintain that fluoride is toxic have a wealth of studies that strongly suggest that they are right. So long as this situation obtains, with neither side willing to give way, there will always be controversy.

References

1. *Responsible science. Ensuring the integrity of the research process.* Vol. I. US Academy of Sciences Panel on Scientific Responsibility and the Conduct of Research. Washington, DC, 1992.
2. Griffiths J. *Covert Action* 1992; 42: 26.
3. Feldman HT, American Board of Allergy and Immunology. Letter to Governor William Milliken's Task Force on Fluoride, 9 May 1979. http://www.ia4u.net/~sherrell/book.html.
4. *Health effects of ingested fluoride.* Subcommittee on Health Effects of Ingested Fluoride, Committee on Toxicology, Board on Environmental Studies and Toxicology, Commission on Life Sciences, US National Research Council, August 1993: 47–8.

33. The UK Review: The Final Word on Fluoride?

> *After 55 years of artificial water fluoridation it is time for opening the scientific debate on this subject. Dentists' dogma and their doctrine that water fluoridation is a safe and effective public health measure can no longer be defended in science.*
> Professor Rudolf Ziegelbecker, 5 August 2000

Publication of the British government White Paper, *Saving Lives: Our Healthier Nation*, seemed an ideal time to settle the fluoridation issue. In 1998, the National Pure Water Association (NPWA) called for an independent public enquiry to examine *all* the evidence on alleged benefits and harm of total fluoride intake from *all* sources, with a view to ending the debate once and for all.

The British government's proposed fundamental change in the fluoridation decision-making process, namely giving responsibility to local councils, was also anticipated by the National Pure Water Association. Suspecting that the government had a hidden agenda, whereby fluoridation would be forced on people, in October 1998 the NPWA flew in Professor A.K. Susheela, a world-renowned authority on fluoridation from the All India Institute of Medical Science, to meet with, and give a presentation to, the Minister for Public Health, Tessa Jowell, and other officials from the Ministry of Health. At the same time, the NPWA presented the Minister with a 30,000-signature petition.

The British government commissions a review

Professor Susheela's presentation appeared to achieve little. The Minister said she had confidence in both her officials and

266

their advisers, one of whom, Dr Waring of the Department of Health, said that experience in the USA, where artificial fluoridation schemes had been in place for over fifty years, provided the necessary evidence of efficacy and safety. The government refused the NPWA request for a full independent inquiry. Instead, it set up an in-house review. It was to be an independent, exhaustive, systematic review of water fluoridation, 'once and for all . . . unchallengeable', said the then Minister of Health, Frank Dobson.

This came as no surprise. Whenever new scientific evidence has threatened fluoride's status, governments of fluoridated countries have immediately appointed a commission or review panel, typically composed of veteran fluoride defenders (no-one opposed to fluoridation has ever been allowed a place on a review panel) to assess the evidence. Such reviews invariably dismiss the new evidence and reaffirm the status quo.

The National Health Service Centre for Reviews and Dissemination (NHSCRD) at the University of York began its work in July 1999. The review panel consisted originally of:

From the NHSCRD, University of York:

Professor Jos Kleijnen (Chairman)
Dr Matthew Bradley
Ms Marijke van Gestel
Kate Misso
Ms Penny Whiting

From the Dental Public Health Unit, Cardiff:

Dr Ivor Chestnutt
Dr Elizabeth Treasure

Later in the process, Dr Bradley left the panel, and Ms Jan Cooper, from the University of Wales Dental School, Cardiff, and Paul Wilson of NHSCRD, joined it. Apart from members from NHSCRD, the only people on this review panel were dentists. You might think this is not unreasonable: after all, isn't fluoride to do with teeth? Well, no. Surely chemicals entering and being incorporated into the body, as fluorides are, fall within the purview of toxicologists. There is no reason whatsoever for any dentists to be on this review panel. Indeed, by their own words in their suggested answer in Chapter 6, they do not consider themselves competent in this matter.

There was also an advisory panel whose members were:

> Professor Trevor Sheldon, York Health Policy Group, University of York (Chairman)
> Earl Baldwin of Bewdley, House of Lords
> Dr Iain Chalmers, UK Cochrane Centre
> Dr Sheila Gibson, Glasgow Homeopathic Hospital
> Ms Sarah Gorin, Help for Health Trust
> Professor M.A. Lennon, Department of Clinical Dental Sciences, University of Liverpool School of Dentistry, Chairman of the British Fluoridation Society
> Dr Peter Mansfield, Director of Templegarth Trust
> Professor J.J. Murray, Dean of Dentistry, University of Newcastle
> Mr Jerry Read, UK Department of Health
> Dr Derek Richards, Centre for Evidence-Based Dentistry
> Professor George Davey Smith, Department of Social Medicine, University of Bristol
> Ms Pamela Taylor, Water UK

Lord Baldwin and Drs Gibson and Mansfield are against water fluoridation. Their inclusion on the advisory panel was to allow a voice to both sides of the debate. The advisory panel, however, could only advise; it would have no say in the final outcome of this review.

A Fluoridation Review Web site was created: it 'aims to keep the public updated on the progress of the review at all stages and to provide them with information on how the review is being conducted, so that the review can be monitored and seen to be free from bias towards either side of the fluoridation debate'.[1]

The review was funded by the National Health Service (known to be in favour of fluoride); three of the review panel's eight members were dentists, one of whom, Elizabeth Treasure, sat on a similar review in New Zealand, which concluded that fluoride was safe; the other five are NHS officials – they work for the organisation that favours fluoridation and that was paying for this review. With such a make-up, this panel did not look either independent or unbiassed. The NHSCRD addressed this point, saying: '[O]ur centre is part of the University of York and is a scientific unit that works independently. We never bow to any pressure towards certain conclusions, because inevitably that will ruin the Centre's prestige, which is high both nationally and internationally. Our output is based on scientifically valid systematic reviews.'

Inclusion (or should that be *exclusion*) criteria

Presumably to ensure that any dangers from fluorides were not missed, the York Review's original protocol stated: 'All studies showing any negative effects from water fluoridation in humans will be considered for inclusion in the review.'[2] And as fluorides are so widespread in modern society, it would consider 'the actual consumption of fluoride from water and **exposure to other sources** of fluorides in the different populations so that the results can be considered in the context of **total fluoride exposure** and that attributable to water supply.'[3] (Emphasis added)

The background to the York Review's draft results stated:

> This study aims to provide a systematic review of the best available evidence of benefits and harm in order to assess the effects of water fluoridation . . .

> Systematic reviews locate, appraise and synthesise evidence from scientific studies in order to provide informative empirical answers to scientific research questions . . . Rather than reflecting the reviews of the authors all being based on only a (possibly biased) selection of the evidence, they aim to contain a comprehensive summary of the available evidence.

At first sight, then, it seemed that the review's deliberations would serve a useful purpose.

But it was not to be. There are tens of thousands of papers on the safety, efficacy and adverse effects of fluoride, yet the review panel managed to locate only 3,246, of which 735 met their relevance criteria and just 214 were included for review. Despite the use of the phrases 'exposure to other sources', 'total fluoride exposure' and 'comprehensive', the protocol for the review excluded all animal studies, all biochemistry studies, all mathematical models and all studies on the effects of fluoride from any source other than artificial water fluoridation. Thus, most of the studies that cast doubt on fluoride, and some that supported it, were deemed unworthy of consideration.

For inclusion, any study had to fulfil the following criteria:

1. **It must be a primary study (i.e. not a review or commentary on existing studies).** Despite admitting that much of the work done on fluoridation is of poor quality, the York Review allowed such early studies but didn't allow the peer-review criticism of their faults. The heavily criticised original study conducted in Kingston and Newburgh, USA, is considered suitable for inclusion. The better-quality later analyses of 1989[4] and 1998,[5] which give a much better idea of the effectiveness or otherwise of fluoridation, are listed in the references, but appear not to have been considered. These studies showed that unfluoridated Kingston had less tooth decay than, and

only half as much dental fluorosis as, fluoridated Newburgh. By not including such data, the York Review panel could only conclude that the fluoridated children were better off – exactly the opposite of the truth.

2. **It must use human subjects; no animal studies will be included in the review.** Just as in other fields of medicine, a great deal of experimental work has been conducted on specially bred animals in laboratory conditions: work that would be impossible on humans for ethical reasons. This criterion ruled out work such as Mullenix's landmark neurotoxicity study.

3. **It must consider fluoridation of public drinking water; studies investigating the effect of fluoride solely from other sources will not be included.** There is so much fluoride in our lives today, even in unfluoridated communities, that excluding the effects from any source other than artificial fluoridation of drinking water was a serious omission that could not fail to distort the findings.

Louis Ronsivalli, for many years laboratory director at the Massachusetts Institute of Technology, and recipient of four US government awards, said of this exclusion:

Because it is ignoring fluoride exposure from all sources, the UK study is, absolutely and without question, being conducted as if by unsupervised schoolchildren. The danger imposed on human health by purposely adding fluoride to public water supplies cannot be scientifically assessed by evaluating only the effect of the fluoride in drinking water supplies. The exclusion of the effects of fluoride from other sources represents the exclusion of relevant variables which must be considered under the scientific rules that must be followed in the conduct of scientific experiments, as well as in the conduct of scientific analyses. Anyone who contends that these variables do not have to be considered, should get into a different line of work. Scientific work is far too important to be conducted by incompetent or careless individuals.

The criteria are narrowed still further

Andreas Schuld is head of a Canadian organisation, Parents of Fluoride-Poisoned Children. Reading through the inclusion criteria and the studies being considered, Schuld noticed that there was not one study on the effects of fluoride on the thyroid gland, although the review panel said it had looked for them. He wrote to the review board, listing a hundred studies that he believed should be included. Dr Matthew Bradley replied:

> Dear Andreas,
> Thank you for your references. We will include them in our assessment of the literature. If you have any other references that are relevant to this review we would be very grateful to receive them. A list of important criteria for the studies is given below:
> All included studies must be:
> Primary studies (no reviews).
> Use human subjects (no animal, or mathematical models).
> Consider fluoridation of public drinking water (no other sources).
> Assess positive and negative effects in humans.
>
> Best wishes
> Matthew Bradley (Research Fellow, NHS CRD)

Schuld replied:

> This is simply unbelievable. I don't mean to be dis-respectful, but it defies all common knowledge regarding

fluorides or other halogens. I live in a nonfluoridated area, and my child suffered from fluoride poisoning from drinking excessive amounts of grape juice, as well as toothpaste use. While it may have been okay 50 years ago to set such a protocol, when fluoride exposure was only a fraction of what it is now, it is simply irresponsible to do so now.

To which Bradley responded:

I understand your concerns, however as you correctly suggest neither I nor CRD as an organisation are in a position to modify the protocol. We have been asked to specifically assess the effect of the fluoridation of public water supplies and therefore can only consider studies designed to meet this objective. To expand the subject matter beyond this would not only go outside our remit but also require extensive resources that are not readily available to us.

We will continue to make the review as open as possible and hope that you will follow the progress of the review via the web interface. We would particularly encourage any comments you would like to make that relate to the review question.

After more correspondence, Schuld was suspicious. He sent this brief e-mail to Dr Bradley:

Hello Matthew,
Would this mean a widening of criteria, or a narrowing?

Andreas

The reply from Dr Bradley was not reassuring:

Thanks for the message Andreas.
I am afraid that, as you may have guessed, it means a narrowing of the criteria.

Shortly after this exchange, Dr Matthew Bradley left the review panel. As he had said, however, the criteria were narrowed, and the wording of several passages was changed to exclude Schuld's evidence:

> Section 4.2. If fluoridation is shown to have beneficial effects, what is the effect over and above that offered by the use of alternative interventions and strategies?

In this section, under 'Participants', the wording was changed subtly, but significantly:

> 1. Populations receiving fluoridated water (either naturally or artificially) who receive fluoride from other identified sources (e.g. food, toothpaste, fluoride tablets, bottled drinks)

was changed to:

> 1. Populations receiving fluoridated water (either naturally or artificially) who receive fluoride from other **artificially supplemented** sources (e.g. food, toothpaste, fluoride tablets, bottled drinks) [emphasis added]

and

> 2. Populations receiving non-fluoridated water who do not receive fluoride from other identified sources

was changed to:

> 2. Populations receiving non-fluoridated water who receive fluoride from other **artificially supplemented** sources [emphasis added]

Under 'Intervention', there were similar changes:

> Fluoride at any concentration present in drinking water and/or fluoride at any concentration provided from sources other than drinking water

was changed to:

> Fluoride at any concentration present in drinking water

This ruled out fluoride from foods, canned drinks, toothpastes, medications, and so on.

The same wording changes were made to Section 4.4: Assessment of the negative health effects of fluoridation.

These changes removed from consideration all sources of fluoride except for those containing artificially added fluoride – and that effectively removed most of the evidence of adverse effects of fluoride in humans.

You absorb more fluoride from a bath

But there remained one glaring omission, which was noticed by George Glasser: the review included no studies addressing the effects of artificially added fluoride that entered the body through the skin. Those who drink artificially fluoridated water will take in 0.40 mg of molecular silicates every day. This is enough to pose a significant risk to health. So, okay, you might think, I will drink only bottled water. But it isn't as simple as that, because drinking water with silicon in it is not the only route by which silicon can enter the body. Research by Glasser and Schuld uncovered the fact that you don't have to drink fluoridated water to be at risk.[6] Both molecular fluorides and silicates are easily absorbed through the skin. By this route they are even more dangerous, as they enter the bloodstream more easily, without the likelihood of being bound in the gut with other minerals from foodstuffs.

As fluoride and silicon are released into the air from clothing and furnishings washed in fluoridated water, you can also inhale them. And this is an even more effective way of getting them inside you than either drinking them or absorbing them through the skin.

The significance of exposures of the skin to contaminants in the environment has been known and accepted for toxicological testing for many years. It is well documented that environmental contaminants such as fluorides are absorbed readily both through the skin and by inhalation.[7]

Studies by Drs H.S. Brown, D.R. Bishop and C.A. Rowan in the early 1980s demonstrated that an average of 64 per cent of the total dose of waterborne contaminants, such as fluoride, are absorbed through the skin.[8] Studies by Dr Julian Andelman, professor of water chemistry, University of Pittsburgh Graduate School of Public Health, also found more chemical exposure from using fluoridated water to wash clothes or take a shower than from drinking it,[9] as absorption through the skin and inhalation directs any contaminants directly into the bloodstream.

The US EPA's own studies confirm these findings. Yet the EPA, as the regulatory agency setting contaminant levels for fluorides in the drinking water, has never commissioned a published study on dermal absorption of fluorides in drinking water,[10] despite applying in 1999 for a grant to research children's vulnerability to toxic substances, because: 'Children have a greater surface area to body weight ratio than adults which may lead to increased dermal absorption.'[11]

So are you going to use bottled water exclusively in the house for everything? Of course not – it's a ridiculous notion.

Fluoride and the thyroid

Between 1932 and 1962, Gorlitzer von Mundy cured hyperthyroidism (overactive thyroid gland) effectively with fluoride baths. Von Mundy warned that such treatment should only be applied to hyperthyroid patients, for to apply such measures to euthyroid (normal) people would surely lead to hypothyroidism (underactive thyroid).[12] It is no surprise, therefore, that hypothyroidism is rising alarmingly in the USA and may now affect as many as 10 per cent of the population.[13]

Young children will often spend from forty-five minutes to two hours playing in the bath. This suggests a significant potential for dermal exposure to waterborne fluorides. Often shampoo, bubble bath and soap are used. Glasser and Schuld point out that almost all bathing products contain sodium lauryl sulphate (SLS) as a foaming agent and that pharmaceutical manufacturers use SLS to increase the absorption of medications used on the skin. SLS added to bath water has been estimated to increase absorption of fluoride from bath water by 9 per cent. SLS is also added to toothpastes, which contain up to 2,500 ppm fluoride. George Glasser believes that it is most significant that no agency in any country that promotes fluoridation of water has ever presented a single study about the most significant route of exposure: the skin.[6]

Hypothyroidism: iodine deficiency or fluoride excess?

According to the WHO, hypothyroidism 'affects 740 million people a year. It causes brain disorders, cretinism, miscarriages and goiter. It is the world's single most important and preventable cause of mental retardation.' In South-east Asia, excluding China, maternal and foetal 'iodine deficiency' is responsible for 101,800 stillbirths and 93,500 neonatal deaths each year.

In 1996 a paper in the *European Journal of Clinical Nutrition* claimed that the high incidence of transient neonatal hypothyroidism in Hong Kong was the result of iodine deficiency.[14] But how can this be? Seafoods, rich in iodine, are eaten extensively in Hong Kong, just as they are throughout South-east Asia. Examination of the iodine content of foodstuffs by the Consumer Council, in association with the Chinese University of Hong Kong, showed that, far from being low, the amount of iodine customarily consumed in a Chinese Hong Kong meal was much *higher* than WHO recommended daily intakes for either children or adults.

Excessive fluoride intake through water, food and air is known to reduce biologically active iodine in the system and cause iodine deficiency. This is the mechanism by which it worked to cure hyperthyroid patients – and at concentrations *lower* than the 'optimal' 1 ppm. Hong Kong's water was fluoridated in 1961. So is the neonatal hypothyroidism really caused by iodine deficiency, or by too much fluoride?

This is another area of research that was excluded from the York Review as a result of the (amended) criteria.

The York Review's objectives and findings

The York Review set out five objectives, or questions to be answered:

1. What effects does fluoridation have on the incidence of dental caries?

This question is fundamental for if there is no benefit, there is no point in fluoridation at all. The Review said: 'To have clear confidence in the ability to answer the question in this objective, the quality of the evidence would need to be higher.' Nevertheless, they did conclude that caries incidence is reduced: '[T]he degree to which it is reduced, however, is not clear from the data available.' But they had excluded recent large-scale and whole-population surveys in such heavily fluoridated countries as Australia,[15] Canada,[16] New Zealand,[17] and the USA,[18] which showed little or no reduction in tooth decay in children's permanent teeth. Tooth decay rates in much of unfluoridated continental Europe, generally lower than in many fluoridated communities, were also excluded.

2. If these effects are beneficial, how do they compare with alternatives to fluoridation?

How can we tell? There is such a huge body of evidence indicating no significant reduction in dental caries in the permanent teeth of children in fluoridated communities compared with unfluoridated communities that there is little point in trying to 'compare' anti-caries effects of water fluoridation with other methods of reducing tooth decay. The review was unable to answer this question satisfactorily.

3. Does fluoridation result in an equitable reduction in caries across groups and different geographical locations?

This question relies on the assumption that there is a benefit from fluoridation, an assumption that is not supported by a substantial body of evidence. British Dental Association figures show that dental caries is similar in areas with and without fluoridation. The Review found that 'the difference between the classes does not vary between the high and low fluoride areas'.

4. Does water fluoridation have negative or adverse health effects?

The review found that there was a direct relationship between fluoride intake and dental fluorosis, with an average 48 per cent affected at levels typically used for water fluoridation.

As fluorosis is indicative of enzyme damage within the tooth, it is clear that other enzymes in the body must be damaged. But exclusion of data such as those submitted by Schuld meant that there was little chance that the review would find damage not normally visible. Nevertheless, it did not find that fluoride does not cause other damage, but said that further, better-quality research is needed.

5. Do natural and artificial water fluoridation differ in their effects?

The review studied a variety of adverse effects but reached no firm conclusion. It stated: 'A wide range of outcomes was considered with many outcomes only discussed in one or two studies. There is thus insufficient evidence for any of these outcomes to compare the effects of artificially and naturally fluoridated water.' But an important aspect of this question is the difference between the chemical used for artificial fluoridation today and what was used previously. The fluorosilicates used in water fluoridation have never been tested. As there are no tests, the York Review could not include them.

In their opening remarks, the review panel members emphasised that this review can be only a part of the evidence that the British government must examine before making a decision to fluoridate the rest of Britain's public water supplies. Nevertheless, the review is being treated by some members of the press as if this is the 'last word' on the fluoridation debate in Britain. It is not. It is not the last scientific word, and it is certainly not the last ethical word.

Peer reviews of the York Review

The combined literature of the York Review and its critics would fill another book. Here are quotes from just three world-renowned scientists who were asked to peer-review the York Review's results, together with quotes from other interested parties:

Paul Connett, PhD, professor of chemistry, St Lawrence University, Canton, New York:

> The York Review's finding that none of these epidemiological studies is worthy of an A grade, underlines the fact that not only is fluoridation a human experiment, the powers that be haven't even done a good job of collecting the data.
>
> The danger of such a review as conducted by the York team is to make everything appear extremely complicated for the ordinary citizen. Let's simplify the picture. No risk is acceptable if it is avoidable. Why take

these risks when based upon the largest study of teeth done in the US the benefit of fluoridation at most represents half a tooth surface saved per child? Why protect the teeth on the outside with a method which has a high chance of damaging them from the inside (dental fluorosis)? Why take these risks when all but three countries in Western Europe do not fluoridate their water and there is no evidence to suggest that their teeth are worse than countries that do? . . . The toxic properties of fluoride are not in dispute.

The York Review has provided enough information for reasonable citizens, scientists and governments to act now. The time has come to end the practice of putting fluoride into drinking water.

Albert W. Burgstahler, PhD, professor emeritus of chemistry, University of Kansas, Lawrence, Kansas, USA:

In considering these objectives and the guidelines laid out for addressing them, one must bear in mind that the DOH is a long-time advocate of fluoridation and is unlikely to retreat from that position.

From a scientific standpoint, the exclusion of animal and laboratory data from the review . . . places undue reliance on admittedly deficient epidemiological investigations that can only be as valid as the adequacy and completeness of the data included in them . . . In terms of human population studies, the omission of all reference to unrefuted peer-reviewed reports of reversible adverse health effects of fluoridation points up a major defect in the review. By not citing pertinent experimental and clinical case-study data on the toxic properties and biomedical hazards of fluoridation, the review clearly has a serious major shortcoming.

Moreover, by not allowing examination of other admittedly important aspects of fluoridation, the DOH has been able to tailor the report to its own restricted views of the subject, thereby making the review very inadequate and misleading in its presentation.

Dr Bruce Spittle, MB, ChB, DPM, FRANZCP, senior lecturer, Department of Psychological Medicine, University of Otago Medical School, Dunedin, New Zealand:

> I have experienced some difficulty in interpreting some of the results . . . After finding some errors I have had doubts about what is accurate and what is not.
>
> I have major reservations about the credibility of the review because of the narrowness of the inclusion criteria and the associated difficulties at looking at the effects of fluoride irrespective of its source using the full range of information available including biochemical and animal studies.

Professor Rudolf Ziegelbecker, PhD, Institute of Environmental Health, Graz, Austria:

> This systematic review of many papers of water fluoridation showed that there is not any paper with evidence of highest level A after 55 years of fluoridation. The level B (evidence of moderate quality) of caries studies, however, is also untenable in view of statistics and natural sciences. I hope that you correct the results of your systematic review and also inform the Department of Health and the public that there is no evidence for 'benefits' of water fluoridation.

Dr Douglas Carnall, British Medical Journal, 7 October 2000:

> The systematic review published this week (p. 855) shows that much of the evidence for fluoridation was derived from low quality studies, that its benefits may have been overstated, and that the risk to benefit ratio

for the development of the commonest side effect (dental fluorosis, or mottling of the teeth) is rather high.

Professionals who propose compulsory preventive measures for a whole population have a different weight of responsibility on their shoulders than those who respond to the requests of individuals for help. Previously neutral on the issue, I am now persuaded by the arguments that those who wish to take fluoride (like me) had better get it from toothpaste rather than the water supply.

George Glasser, US investigative journalist specialising in pollution:

> While almost every credible governmental and international health agency specifically states that dermal and inhalation exposures are significant in determining the overall potential lifetime exposure of the individual, the NHS Centre for Reviews and Dissemination at York University failed to acknowledge the present criteria for research methodology in the fluoridation review.
>
> Many observers, including this writer, who investigate current scientific review criteria will dismiss the York review on the basis that the panels did not address all modes of exposure, and most importantly, the special children's issues.

E.M. Vaughan, on behalf of the directors, National Pure Water Association Ltd.:

> The National Pure Water Association Ltd. expresses its deep disappointment that the criteria for selection of research papers were seriously restrictive.
>
> We are particularly critical of the exclusion of all existing animal studies, exposure via dermal absorption

and the biochemistry of fluoride exposure from sources other than drinking water. Nor did the Review consider the total exposure of human populations to toxic fluorides, which essentially determines the severity of adverse health effects.

NPWA Ltd. regrets that this Review represents a missed opportunity to explore the breadth of fluoride research. Whatever the Final Report may conclude, the self-evident deficiencies of this Review compromise the security of the NHS CRD's findings.

Andreas Schuld, Parents of Fluoride-Poisoned Children:

Fluorides are the worst endocrine disruptor imaginable . . . What was once known as the fluoride–iodine antagonism can now be explained in detail by thousands of papers showing the fluoride power on G-protein activation . . . Experiments with rats clearly show that the amounts required to cause thyroid disturbance are identical to the levels which have been identified to cause dental fluorosis.

Health care providers in those areas need to be properly informed how to deal with the effects of this fluoride poisoning. This is an urgent global concern.

Saying that the York Review might well turn out be the greatest scientific fraud ever undertaken by a centre in charge of evaluating scientific information in the interest of public health, Schuld urged 'the people in the UK to ask for an immediate public inquiry into the scientific misconduct clearly prevalent at the York Center'.

The Review's findings are misinterpreted

British Minister of Health, Yvette Cooper, used the result of this review as a basis for recommending more water fluoridation.

'We will be encouraging health authorities with high levels of dental decay to consider fluoridating their water as part of their overall oral health strategy,' she said. 'The report of the evidence review will help ensure that local decisions are based on an authoritative, readily accessible summary of research into the safety and efficacy of water fluoridation.'[19]

The British Fluoridation Society also uses the York Review's findings on its Questions and Answers Web page to support its call for more fluoridation.[20] The BFS says:

Q1. What are the findings of the review?

- The review was set up to establish whether fluoridation is still effective, and whether it is still safe, and the report is unequivocal: water fluoridation is EFFECTIVE and SAFE.

- The review findings in relation to general health effects are unequivocal: there is no association between water fluoride and any adverse health effect . . .

- Importantly, the review also confirms that water fluoridation reduces inequalities in dental health. It narrows the dental health gap between young children living in poverty and their more affluent peers.

Q5. What does the review say about dental fluorosis?

- The review recognises dental fluorosis as a cosmetic issue, not a health problem, and acknowledges that it occurs in non-fluoridated as well as fluoridated areas.

Q16. How can the government take forward this measure now?

- On the basis of the findings of the York Review the government should now press ahead with its plans to 'introduce a legal obligation on water companies to fluoridate where there is strong local support for doing so'.

And an editorial in the *British Dental Journal* said:

> The researchers also found evidence that water fluoridation reduces inequalities in dental health by narrowing the dental health gap between young children living in poverty and their more affluent peers. They found no evidence to support claims that water fluoridation caused any harm. On fluorosis, they estimate that fluoridation would slightly increase the prevalence of dental fluorosis of 'aesthetic concern'. Finally they found no difference between naturally and artificially fluoridated water.[21]

But these are gross misinterpretations. Professor Trevor Sheldon refuted them in the following statement:[22]

> From: Department of Health Studies,
> Innovative Centre, York Science Park,
> University Road, York, Y010 5DG
> 10 December 2000
>
> In my capacity of chair of the Advisory Group for the systematic review on the effects of water fluoridation recently conducted by the NHS Centre for Reviews and Dissemination the University of York and as its founding director, I am concerned that the results of the review have been widely misrepresented . . . It is particularly worrying then that statements which mislead the public about the review's findings have been made in press releases and briefings by the British Dental Association, the National Alliance for Equity in Dental Health and the British Fluoridation Society. I should like to correct some of these errors.
>
> 1. Whilst there is evidence that water fluoridation is effective at reducing caries, the quality of the studies was generally moderate and the size of the

estimated benefit, only of the order of 15%, is far from 'massive'.

2. The review found water fluoridation to be significantly associated with high levels of dental fluorosis which was not characterised as 'just a cosmetic issue'.

3. The review did not show water fluoridation to be safe. The quality of the research was too poor to establish with confidence whether or not there are potentially important adverse effects in addition to the high levels of fluorosis. The report recommended that more research was needed.

4. There was little evidence to show that water fluoridation has reduced social inequalities in dental health.

5. The review could come to no conclusion as to the cost-effectiveness of water fluoridation or whether there are different effects between natural or artificial fluoridation.

6. Probably because of the rigour with which this review was conducted, these findings are more cautious and less conclusive than in most previous reviews.

7. The review team was surprised that in spite of the large number of studies carried out over several decades there is a dearth of reliable evidence with which to inform policy. Until high quality studies are undertaken providing more definite evidence, there will continue to be legitimate scientific controversy over the likely effects and costs of water fluoridation.

(Signed) T.A. Sheldon,
Professor Trevor Sheldon, MSc, DSc, FMedSci

Conclusion

In 1985 Professor Phillipe Grandjean, professor of environmental medicine at the University of Odense, Denmark, wrote to the US Environmental Agency about a WHO study on fluorine and fluoride. He pointed out:

> Information which could cast any doubt on the advantage of fluoride supplements was left out by the Task Group. Unless I had been present myself, I would have found it hard to believe.

The same can be said of the York Review. One is now left to wonder why the Review was conducted. If this review was worth a year's work by so many highly paid 'scientists' and government officials; if it was worth spending scarce NHS money on; if it was really to be a 'once and for all, unchallengeable' examination of the benefits and adverse effects of fluoridation, why were the inclusion criteria manipulated to exclude pertinent data?

Despite the narrowness of the initial inclusion criteria and the subsequent shifting of the goalposts, the review panel was not able to provide a definitive answer about the safety and effectiveness of fluoridation. The panel admits that all the evidence considered was of poor quality and may well have been biassed.

There is no doubt that the York Review and the spin put on it by government and pro-fluoridationists has been a source of disappointment to, and has provoked extreme scepticism in, those who had hoped to see some definitive assessment of fluoride's health role. The effect of the final report can probably be summed up best by Lord Baldwin, another member of the advisory panel. He writes in his comments on the York Review:

> The findings are capable of spinning in either direction, and it is worth getting a copy of the full report.

The reviewers make clear that they cannot answer the question whether to fluoridate or not, since this involves questions of ethics, ecology, cost-effectiveness and law, as well as total fluoride exposure from sources other than water, which were outside their brief. They stress that benefits must be set against harmful effects in coming to decisions.

The following five statements are incontrovertible.

1. There are no high-quality studies in the water fluoridation literature. All are of moderate to low quality, with a moderate to high risk of bias, which means that *no* answer to *any* of the questions can be given with full confidence, and some of them are given with little if any confidence at all. This is surprising in view of the claims made for fluoridation. The evidence for evening out dental inequalities between social classes – a frequently made claim – is so weak as to be highly speculative.

2. The quantity of evidence is also thin, especially for the benefits, the benefits over and above other anti-caries measures, caries comparisons across social groups, differences (if any) between natural and artificial fluoridation, and dangers other than for fluorosis, bone fractures/disorders, and cancer.

3. The best evidence, though it is not good, is for benefits in caries reduction (less than previously believed), and dental fluorosis (more). It is possible, though not very likely, that either or both of these findings could be due to bias or other confounding factors.

4. Numbers who may benefit from fluoridation appear to match the numbers who get fluorosed

teeth. A figure of 48% of people fluorosed at 1 ppm is surprisingly high (the *British Medical Journal* considers this an overestimate, though they may not be right). Although only c. 1 in 4 of those with fluorosis have seriously unsightly teeth, dental fluorosis is recognised by the DoH as a sign of systemic toxicity and not simply a cosmetic effect.

5. The review team were not allowed to make policy recommendations, which the DoH saw as its own responsibility. Nevertheless the report concluded with suggestions for further research which it felt to be necessary:

   (a) The long-term benefits for adult teeth should be assessed, i.e. not just studies on children, and any such studies should look for adverse effects at the same time (these may take longer to show themselves than present research has allowed for), and could also look for social class effects;

   (b) More research is needed into possible adverse effects;

   (c) All future research should be of high quality, using proper methodology to control for confounding factors such as total fluoride exposure, sugar consumption, erupted teeth, blinding of observers, and spending on dental health.

   It should also look formally at lower concentrations of fluoride such as 0.8 ppm.

Beyond the above findings of the review, which in the opinion of experts is seen as among the best scientific examples of its kind in its thoroughness, care and openness, it is a matter of opinion whether the evidence presented supports a policy of general water fluoridation. One view, shared by some of the independent scientists involved in the review, is that a public health measure which treats whole populations must be founded on impeccable science, and that on the basis of the evidence presented there is no good case for fluoridation. Anyone who considers this report to be a ringing endorsement of water fluoridation is either dishonest, a fanatic, or scientifically illiterate.

The government's York Review, indeed all research conducted on drinking water fluoridation, was concerned only with direct oral ingestion from water, using either calcium or sodium fluoride. No research has ever been carried out on the chronic effects of exposure to fluorosilicates, whether they be in water, food or air, and none seems likely while 'reviews' restrict their examinations to the effects produced by the addition of sodium fluoride to water alone. Any claims that these substances are safe or efficacious are specious.

The British government's White Paper on health, *Saving Lives: Our Healthier Nation*, specifically stated that this review would examine the effects of fluoride on health. It didn't.

The title the NHSCRD dreamed up for their press release was 'The final word on fluoride'. It isn't.

References

1. http://www.york.ac.uk/inst/crd/fluoinc.htm
2. http://www.york.ac.uk/inst/crd/fluofaq.htm
3. http://www.york.ac.uk/inst/crd/fluorid4.htm
4. Kumar JV, Green EL, Wallace W, Carnahan T. Trends in dental fluorosis and dental caries prevalences in Newburgh and Kingston, NY. *Am J Public Health* 1989; 79: 565–9.
5. Kumar JV, Swango PA, Lininger LL et al. Changes in dental fluorosis and dental caries in Newburgh and

Kingston, New York. *Am J Public Health* 1998; 88: 1866–70.

6. Glasser G, Schuld A. Your child's vulnerability to toxic substances in the environment. *Fluoride Watershed* June 2000 6 (1).

7. *Prevention, pesticides and toxic substances* (7101). EPA 712-C-96–350, June 1996. Health effects test guidelines, OPPTS 870.7600, 870.7600: Dermal penetration; EPA, *Exposure factors handbook*, August 1996: 'Factors that affect dermal exposure are the express way in which a combined amount of material comes into contact with the skin; the dose–response relationship to calculate risk and the rate at which the contaminant is absorbed; the body weight to be used in the exposure calculations; and the exposure duration'; *Dermal exposure assessment: Principles and applications*, EPA/600/8-91/011B, January 1991.

8. Brown HS, Bishop DR, Rowan CA. American Chemical Society Meeting, Anaheim, CA, USA, *Am J Publ Hlth* 1984; 74: 479–84.

9. Andelman J. Non-ingestion exposure to chemicals in potable water. Working paper 84–03, University of Pittsburgh, 1984.

10. *Dermal exposure assessment: Principals and applications*. EPA/600/8-91/011B, January 1991.

11. *Children's vulnerability to toxic substances in the environment*. Science to Achieve Results Program: 1999 Research Grants. National Center for Environmental Research and Quality Assurance USEPA.

12. von Mundy G. Einfluss von Fluor und Jod auf den Stoffwechsel, insbesondere auf die Schilddrüse. *Münch Med Wochenschrift* 1963; 105: 234–47.

13. Canaris GJ, Manowitz NR, Mayor G, Ridgway EC. The Colorado Thyroid Disease Prevalence Study. *Arch Intern Med* 2000; 160: 526–34.

14. Kung AWC, Chan LWL, Low LCK, Robinson JD. Existence of iodine deficiency in Hong Kong – a coastal city in southern China. *Eur J Clin Nutr* 1996; 50: 8.

15. Diesendorf M. A re-examination of Australian fluoridation trials. *Search* 1986; 17: 256–61.

16. Gray AS. Fluoridation: Time for a new base line? *J Can Dent Assoc* 1987; 53: 763–5.

17. Colquhoun J. Fluorides and the decline in tooth decay in New Zealand. *Fluoride* 1993; 26: 125–34. Cf. *Community Health Studies* 1987; 11: 85–90; *Community Health Studies* 1988; 12: 187–91.

18. Hildebolt CF, Elvin-Lewis M, Molnar S et al. Caries prevalences among geochemical regions of Missouri. *Am J Phys Anthropol* 1989; 78: 79–92; Yiamouyiannis JA. Water fluoridation and tooth decay: Results from the 1986–1987 national survey of US schoolchildren. *Fluoride* 1990; 23: 55–67; Steelink C. Letter. *Chem Eng News* 17 July 1992: 2–3; Cf. Abstract of AAAS presentation: An analysis of the causes of tooth decay in children in Tucson, Arizona. *Fluoride* 1994; 27: 238.

19. *Hansard*, 30 Oct 2000: Column: 243W.

20. http://www.derweb.co.uk/bfs/york_qa.html. Accessed 23 December 2000.

21. Grace M. Facts on fluoridation. *Br Dent J* 2000; 189: 405.

22. York Review Chairman concerned about 'misrepresentation' by profluoride lobby. http://www.npwa.freeserve.co.uk/sheldon_letter.html.

34. Are You at Risk?

> There's nothing like a glass of cool, clear water to quench one's thirst. But the next time you or your child reaches for one, you might want to question whether that water is, in fact, too toxic to drink. If your water is fluoridated, the answer may well be yes.
> Gary Null, PhD

Ireland

All cities and most towns in Ireland, covering about 75 per cent of the population, are served with fluoridated water: thus most are at risk. Your water supply company can tell you whether you are one of the lucky few who are not. They can also tell you what the fluoride content is if you live in a fluoridated area.

Despite the forum on fluoridation, there are plans to extend fluoridation to the following areas as soon as possible:

North Western Health Board

- Ballyshannon, Fanad East and West, Lough Inn, West Inishowen, The Pollen Dam, County Donegal
- North County Sligo region

Midwestern Health Board

- North County Clare region
- Croom, County Limerick

South Eastern Health Board

- Kilmacthomas, Ballyduff, County Waterford
- Fardystown, County Wexford
- Hacketstown, County Carlow
- Coalbrook/Ballincurry, Graigue and Glengurra, County Tipperary

Southern Health Board

- Youghal UDC, Bula Treatment Plant, County Cork
- Brosna/Knocknagoshel, County Kerry

North Eastern Health Board

- Athboy, County Meath
- Virginia, County Cavan
- Clontibret, County Monaghan

Eastern Regional Health Authority

- The Curragh, County Kildare

Midland Health Board

- Martinstown, County Westmeath

Britain

Many people believe that all British tap water is fluoridated. This is not so. Scotland and Wales are not fluoridated at all (yet), and only about 9 per cent of people in England live in areas where drinking water is polluted with fluoride. You are one of those people only if you live in one of the following postal districts:

These districts have naturally occurring calcium fluoride in their water at more than 0.5 ppm:
    Durham: DH1, DH2; part of DH6
    Essex: CO1–6, CO8–10
    Lincolnshire: Part of LN13
    Peterborough: PE2, PE4
    Suffolk: IP1–8, IP13, IP14, IP28–30, IP33
    Teesside: TS27, TS28
    Tyneside: NE25, NE26, NE29; part of NE30

These districts have artificially fluoridated drinking water:
    Berkshire: RG1, RG4–6, RG40, RG41

Birmingham: B6–11, B13–21, B23–34, B37, B40, B42, B45, B60–62, B65–71; parts of Central Birmingham and B36, B38, B43, B44, B46, B47, B63, B64, B90, B92, B97

Buckinghamshire: Parts of SG18, SG19

Chelmsford: CM1

Coventry: CV1–6, CV10, CV11; parts of CV 7–9, CV12, CV13

Crewe: Parts of CW1, CW2, CW5–7, CW12, CW17

Cumbria: CA24, CA25, CA27, CA28

Dartford: DA1

Derbyshire: DE13–15

Doncaster: DN15, DN16, DN18–21, DN38–40; parts of DN9, DN10, DN17, DN22, DN31, DN37

Dudley: Parts of DY6, DY9, DY10

Durham: DH2, DH7–9; parts of DH15

Kent, around Ashford: TN26

Lancaster: Parts of LA19

Leicestershire: Parts of LE10 and LE18

Lincolnshire: LN1, LN2, LN4–7

Milton Keynes: MK17, MK43–46

Nottinghamshire: NG18–20; parts of NG17, NG21–24, NG31, NG32 and NG34

Oxfordshire: Part of OX9

Sheffield: Parts of S80

Shrewsbury: Parts of SY13, SY14

Stoke: Parts of ST7, ST8

Tonbridge: TN26

Tyneside: NE1–6, NE8, NE12, NE15–18, NE21, NE23, NE25–27, NE39, NE42, NE43, NE45, NE46; parts of NE9–11, NE13, NE19, NE20, NE24, NE28, NE44, NE46–48, NE65

Walsall, Wolverhampton: WV2, WV3, WV13, WV14; parts of WV6–8

Warwickshire: There may be fluoridated areas in the south of the county.

Worcestershire: Parts of WR7, WR9–11

Contact your local water authority for analysis figures of your tap water's fluoride content. They are legally obliged to give you this information and, in my experience, are very willing to do so.

If your water contains more than 0.4 ppm, your only recourse (other than to complain to your water supply company) is to install a water purification system that removes fluoride. Note, however, that most water filters do not remove fluoride. Fluoride is not removed by boiling, home water-softening systems, sediment filters or ultraviolet systems. Carbon filtration systems alone will not remove fluoride from the water, although carbon filtration units that contain activated alumina can reduce the amount. Fluoride removal can be achieved either by distillation or by using a reverse osmosis system. Depending on the size and the type of the system, it will remove between 90 and 99 per cent of the fluoride in the water.[1]

A suitable filter may be purchased from the following companies:

- Ecowater, Mill Road, Stokenchurch, High Wycombe, Bucks, HP14 3TP
- Fresh Water Filters Co. Ltd., Carlton House, Aylmere Road, Leytonstone, London, E11 3AD
- Crouch Water Softener Services, 631 London Road, Westcliffe-on-Sea, Essex, SS0 9PE

Minimising the risk from fluoride

Fluoride is the thirteenth most abundant element, so it is impossible to remove it all. But you can reduce the risk of getting an overdose by taking the following precautions.

- Avoid anything that you know contains fluoride.

- Use fluoride-free toothpaste: Boot's Non-Fluoride, Tom's, Tea Tree, Sarakan, Kingfisher Natural Propolis,

Weleda, Aloedent and shops' own brands are available from supermarkets, pharmacies and health-food shops.

- Eat foods low in fluoride: milk, eggs, red meats (not organ meats), fruit with a protective rind (watermelon, orange, banana, coconut), fruits packed in their own juices (pineapple) and those canned in non-fluoridated or low-fluoridated countries.

- Peel apples and grapes before eating, and avoid apple and grape juice. Apples and grapes are commonly sprayed with high-fluoride cryolite pesticides. The fluoride stays in the fruits' skin and is incorporated into juices and wines.

- Avoid all canned drinks and canned produce from fluoridated countries: the USA, Ireland, Canada, Australia and New Zealand.

- Avoid wines and other drinks from fluoridated countries.

- Don't drink tea without milk: tea contains between 4.4 and 12 ppm of fluoride. Just one cup can be enough for an overdose. The calcium in milk mitigates the effects of fluoride.

- Stay away from areas that fluoridate water supplies (see list above for UK areas).

- If you live in a fluoridated area, do not use aluminium cookware.

- Avoid using non-stick kitchenware: non-stick coatings, such as Teflon and Tefal, are made of fluoride. Scrapes and other damage can release a significant amount of fluoride into food. Non-stick coatings are usually applied to aluminium pans. This combination increases the risk enormously even if you do not live in a fluoridated area.

- Avoid drugs containing fluoride: if you are taking any of the following, contact your doctor for a fluoride-free alternative.

  - Prozac (fluoxetine)
  - Rohypnol (flunitrazepam)
  - Diflucan (fluconazole)
  - Flixonase or Flixotide (fluticasone)
  - Stelazine (trifluoperazine)
  - Fluanxol or Depixol (flupenthixol)
  - Floxapen (flucloxacillin)
  - Asthma drugs that use propellants containing fluoride: Ventolin and Becotide

- Take vitamin B6 and C supplements. These minimise the effects of fluoride.

- Take supplements of calcium and magnesium salts to help reduce fluoride absorption from the stomach and assist in elimination.

- Maintain good general and dental health with meat, dairy products, varied vegetables, fresh fruits and pulses. Reduce intakes of starches (bread, pasta, cereals, rice) and sugars.

Symptoms of fluoride toxicity are similar to those for hypothyroid. If your symptoms are caused by fluoride, you should notice a marked improvement within days or weeks. And symptoms will return once you are re-exposed to a source of fluoride.

The following can test for fluoride poisoning:
- Biolab Medical Unit, 9 Weymouth Street, London, W1N 3FF

For a test on fluoride sensitivity and white-cell depression:
- British Fluoridation Exposure Group, PO Box 5484, Leicester, LE3 3WH

For a test measuring 24-hour urine output of fluoride, contact:

- Dr Peter Mansfield, Templegarth Trust, PO Box 6, Louth, Lincs., LN11 8XL

... and a banana to finish?

Incidentally, the international news magazine *Newsweek*, reported that French scientists are currently working on a genetically modified banana capable of fighting tooth decay. Jos Bov, a former director of the National Institute for Agronomic Research in Bordeaux, says, 'In some African countries where they may not have the money to buy toothpaste, why not eat a transgenic banana that will prevent cavities instead?'[2]

I wonder if they will engineer fluoride into it?

Reference

1. Proceedings of the International Conference on Fluorides, 21–24 March 1989, Pine Mountain, Georgia, USA, *J Dent Res* (Special Issue), February 1990: 69.
2. 'Like father, like son', *Newsweek*, 5 February 2001: 28.

35. Conclusion

A long habit of not thinking a thing wrong, gives it a superficial appearance of being right.
Thomas Paine, *Introduction to Common Sense*, 1776

No scientist is infallible and every scientist is entitled to his errors. But when he omits crucial facts in order to influence laymen, he does not become a dishonest scientist; he ceases to be a scientist.
Professor Petr Beckman

The philosophy behind the 'search for truth' by the proponents of water fluoridation is well illustrated by the famous Sufi story about Mullah Nasrudin, an enlightened, fabled teacher. While on his hands and knees, peering on the street for a lost key, he was approached by a friend.

'You lost your key here, Mullah?' his friend enquired.

'No,' said Nasrudin, 'I lost it in my house.'

'Then why are you looking here?' asked his friend.

'Because', said Nasrudin, 'the light is better here.'

Integrity in science

'The keystone of professional conduct is integrity,' says the National Association of Environmental Professionals' Code of Ethics and Standards of Practice for Environmental Professionals (USA). What this means, among other things, is that professionals are responsible for the truth of their work, which must be conducted without 'dishonesty, fraud, deceit or misrepresentation or discrimination'. It also means that they must not allow bias to twist facts or conclusions to ensure a preconceived or desired outcome. But their responsibility does not cease when a paper is published: they must also ensure that it is not misrepresented by others, or altered to change its data or meaning.

When fluoridation was first proposed, individual fluoride intake was determined to be less than 1 mg per day. That is no longer the case. We could be charitable and accept that the original dental and public health promoters might not have anticipated that their actions would raise total fluoride levels to their present high values, or that in their haste to initiate the artificial addition of fluoride to drinking water, they failed to carry out the projections required to predict the consequences.

Fluoridation promoters consider the increased numbers of fluoridated communities 'progress' along the path to a society that will, ultimately, be freed from tooth decay. Those who are familiar with the historical development of the concept of fluoridation and the evidence of its lack of effectiveness and of its adverse effects on teeth, the skeletal system and soft tissues, must disagree. While lack of adequate information sixty years ago may excuse mistakes of the past, failure to learn from these mistakes and take appropriate action could now be interpreted as negligence.

Proceed with caution

The 'precautionary principle' has become an established argument in debates on the environment and health. There are various definitions, but in essence the principle says: If in doubt, err on the side of caution. If this principle were to be applied to fluoridation, it would be stopped tomorrow (if not yesterday). Instead, studies invariably conclude: 'We're not sure, more studies are needed. In the meantime, the evidence is not strong enough to stop fluoridation.' This is doing things the wrong way round. If there is doubt about the effects of fluoridation, then it should be stopped, to be restarted only if and when research indicates that it is safe, effective and ethically defensible.

A growing number of scientists, dentists and activists assert that the United States has a large-scale public health disaster on its hands. There are even those in the dental profession who call for 'a new baseline' or a 'change in traditional thinking' and point to the general acceptance in continental Europe that the systemic use of fluoride to prevent dental caries is passé. There has also been an obvious switch on the part of the American Dental Association elite away from a 'structural' to a 'remineralisation' rationale. Despite this, orthodoxy regarding fluoridation remains entrenched in the USA, Canada, Ireland and the United Kingdom.

In most medical research, the course follows a recognised pattern: a scientist has an idea and formulates a hypothesis. If it is thought plausible and worthwhile, studies and trials are set up to confirm or refute that hypothesis. If those studies confirm the hypothesis, all well and good. If they do not confirm the hypothesis, then the hypothesis is revised to fit the evidence provided by the studies, or it is rejected as unproven.

In the case of fluoride, however, a different philosophy obtains. If the studies and trials do not support the fluoride hypothesis (and they don't), the fluoride hypothesis remains sound, and it is the follow-up confirmatory research that must be at fault. But water fluoridation has been practised for over half a century. During that time, as the York Review admits, there have been no properly conducted studies proving indisputably that fluoride is beneficial, and considerable doubt remains about the safety and efficacy of water fluoridation.

Fluoridation, especially in the United States, has been established as a 'national goal' or 'mission'. Billions of US taxpayers' dollars have been spent over the past fifty years to fulfil this mission – not only in the USA, but in other countries too, including Britain and Ireland. As is typical of so many government-sponsored endeavours, this mission will continue even though there is ample evidence that the fluoride–caries hypothesis is invalid and that fluoridation has created a major public health problem: endemic fluorosis. And in spite of the fact that fluoridation poses a definite threat to the environment.

The public is already against fluoridation and is increasingly likely to call for a halt to the programme when evidence emerges that:

- Dental fluorosis is not merely cosmetic but is a sign that we have poisoned our children.

- The adverse effects of fluoride are well-founded, especially when total fluoride intake is considered.

- Fluoridation is a failure and is costing us dearly in terms of treatment for adverse effects and losses in the ecosystem due to fluoride pollution.

- Fluoridation is a gross misuse of increasingly scarce healthcare resources.

There is a disturbing bias on the part of many in the research community to search only for 'positive' results. These, especially when they concern human health, are more likely than 'negative' findings to be accepted, true or not.

Once the idea that '1 ppm fluoride, artificially added to drinking water, prevents dental caries' became accepted, only those studies supporting or enhancing it were acceptable. There had to be something wrong with research that produced results that were contrary. The early trials are a graphic example of research that was 'at fault'. Whether intentionally or through ineptitude, arrogance or ignorance of scientific method, the early research of Dean and others is an example of manipulating the results to obtain positive support for the hypotheses underlying fluoridation.

Some defenders have intimated that these trials were not meant to be scientific studies comparing a fluoridated population with controls but were merely demonstrations that fluoride could be added to the water supply without any immediate mechanical problems or apparent adverse effects. Such is the quicksand upon which the whole fluoridation edifice is built.

Like any commercial product, fluoridation has been advertised and promoted over the past half-century to the point where to millions it is 'the truth'. The companies manufacturing and marketing dental products commission their own research and fund dental meetings on the subject. The list of corporate sponsors of an international conference held in Pine Mountain, Georgia, USA, in 1989 included many familiar names: Cheesebrough–Ponds; Unilever; Johnson & Johnson; Procter & Gamble; Colgate–Palmolive; Bristol Myers; and others.[1]

And they are not the only ones with an interest in fluoride: the Princeton Resource Center publishes a magazine for dentists. This has nothing to do with the university of the same name – it is financed by the confectionery manufacturer M&M/Mars. Also in the background, letting these companies work for them, are those industries that supply the raw materials used for fluoridation or that benefit from fluoride's benign image. Without fluoridation, millions of tons of hexafluorosilicic acid would have to be funnelled into holding ponds and treated at great expense. Instead, it is used to turn a profit.

This relentless promotion of fluoride as a 'dental benefit', and refusal to listen to any who say otherwise, is responsible for the huge neglect in proper assessment of its toxicity, an issue that has become a major concern for many nations. There is no substance as biochemically active in living organisms as fluoride. Uncontrolled consumption of fluoridated compounds might well be contributing to many modern diseases currently afflicting mankind, particularly those involving thyroid dysfunction. As the toxicity of fluoride is undisputed, why are its adverse effects disputed?

This myopic mentality also means that the real causes of dental caries are not addressed.

The truth, now becoming increasingly evident, is that fluoridation, and the proclaimed benefit of fluoride as a way of preventing dental decay, may well turn out to be the greatest scientific fraud ever perpetrated upon an unsuspecting public, a fraud perpetrated by a supposedly caring profession whose philosophy is arrogant and based entirely on the ignorance of its members.

Reference

1. Proceedings of the International Conference on Fluorides, 21–24 March 1989, Pine Mountain, GA, USA. *J Dent Res* (Special Issue), February 1990: 69.

Appendix A

Scientific Opposition to Fluoride

In addition to the scientists who have lost their jobs and been vilified for speaking out against fluoride, as described in Chapter 19, there are many more who have voiced their concerns. The list given below is far from exhaustive. These men and women were chosen because they are leaders and respected members of their professions, with impeccable credentials in science, dentistry, medicine and law.

Dentists

John Colquhoun, BDS, MPhil, PhD, DipEd. Former principal dental officer, Auckland; Department of Education, University of Auckland, New Zealand:

> When the socioeconomic variable is allowed for, child dental health appears to be better in the unfluoridated areas.[1]

David C. Kennedy, DDS. Professor and past president, International Academy of Oral Medicine and Toxicology:

> During the Fountain Congressional hearings of 1977, the NCI admitted that they had relied upon no scientific data whatsoever when they claimed 25 years earlier that fluoride would be safe to add to the community water supplies.[2]

Hardy Limeback, DDS, PhD. Professor of preventive dentistry, University of Toronto:

Children under three should never use fluoridated toothpaste or drink fluoridated water. And baby formula must never be made up using [fluoridated] Toronto tap water. Never.[3]

Don MacAuley (see Chapter 6).

George E. Meinig, DDS. Founding member, American Association of Endodontics:

Opposing this issue was difficult enough without having to buck slandering tactics by colleagues. Even worse, in the eyes of the public, a dentist that didn't support fluoridation, appeared to favour people having cavities in order to increase personal income. Why, then, did a few prevention-minded dentists and physicians face the wrath and indignation of both the public and professionals? There are substantial scientific reasons.[4]

Tohru Murakami, DDS, PhD. Vice-president, Japanese Society for Fluoride Research, Japan:

I just shudder to think how many cases of fluoride poisoning have been covered up by false science.[5]

Philip R.N. Sutton, DDSc, FRACDS. Former senior lecturer in dental science, University of Melbourne:

The fifty-year-old fluoridation hypothesis has not been confirmed. Despite this, millions of people are still medicated with fluoride by government decree, on the assumption that this process has been proved to be entirely safe, and very efficacious in reducing dental caries. In fact, the scientific basis of fluoridation is very unsatisfactory. It is promoted, in the main, by emotion-based 'endorsements' rather than by scientifically acceptable evidence.[6]

Scientists and prominent people in other specialisations

Judge Beatrice J. Brown, Brattleboro, Vermont:

> As a judge who has to run for office every two years,
> and have [*sic*] since my election in 1948, had to defeat
> six men lawyers to retain it, I should be by now
> sufficiently a politician to realize that I may be
> jeopardizing my office at the next election if I oppose
> fluoridation, but my conscience does not allow me to
> remain silent on the issue when I see such ignorance as
> to the physical effects of fluoride and blind acceptance
> of it as a measure made in Heaven itself for the benefit
> of our children.[7]

Albert W. Burgstahler, PhD (Organic Chemistry and
Environmental Fluoride). Professor of Chemistry, University
of Kansas:

> In view of the extensive evidence contradicting contrary
> claims based to a considerable degree on flawed
> research, mandatory addition of industrial waste
> fluoride (from the phosphate fertilizer industry) to
> public water supplies clearly requires careful scrutiny
> and at present can hardly be seen as justified or
> desirable.[2]

Dean Burk, PhD (Biochemistry). Former senior chemist and
director, Cytochemistry Section, National Cancer Institute:

> Everything causes cancer? Perhaps. Conceivably even a
> single electron at the other side of the universe. The real
> question is, how likely is any one particular cause? In
> point of fact, fluoride causes more human cancer death,
> and causes it faster, than any other chemical.[7]

Robert J. Carton, PhD (Environmental Sciences and Risk
Assessment). Former risk assessment manager for the Office
of Toxic Substances, US Environmental Protection Agency:

The fluoride in drinking water standard, or Recommended Maximum Contaminant Level (RMCL), published by EPA in the *Federal Register* on Nov. 14, 1985, is a classic case of political interference with science. The regulation is a fraudulent statement by the Federal Government that 4 milligrams per litre (mg/l) of fluoride in drinking water is safe with an adequate margin of safety. There is evidence that critical information in the scientific and technical support documents used to develop the standard was falsified by the Department of Health and Human Services and the Environmental Protection Agency to protect a long-standing public health policy.[8]

Paul Connett, PhD (Environmental Chemistry and Toxicology). Professor of chemistry, St Lawrence University, Canton, New York:

A very powerful lobby has attempted to put the fluoridation debate off-limits. After our extensive reading of the arguments on both sides we believe the debate is off-limits because fluoridation is a house of cards waiting to fall . . . the argument for fluoridating the public's water supply – the reduction of dental caries for children under the age of twelve (hardly life-threatening) – is hugely outweighed by the many potential health hazards, some of which are extremely serious indeed.[9]

Mark Diesendorf, BSc, PhD. Director, Institute for Sustainable Futures, University of Technology, Sydney, Australia:

A review of recent scientific literature reveals a consistent pattern of evidence – hip fractures, skeletal fluorosis, the effect of fluoride on bone structure, fluoride levels in bones and osteosarcomas – pointing to the existence of causal mechanisms by which fluoride damages bones.[10]

C.G. Dobbs. Professor of microbiology, University of North Wales, associate of the Royal College of Science, formerly at King's College London:

> [Fluoridation] is of doubtful legality; it offends deep convictions concerning doctoring without consent; it is against the medical tradition of care for the individual; against the function of a public water supply; against sane economics; against the considered opinion of eminent nutritionists, biochemists, physiologists, pharmacologists, allergists, toxicologists; above all, it is against natural caution and common sense.[2]

Gregory Erickson, RS, CHO. Director of Public Health, Wilmington, Massachusetts:

> This pattern of a higher crude death rate in the cities with fluoridated water supplies was apparent for all categories of death except for those by accidental means and suicide.[11]

Ben F. Feingold, MD (Physician). Chief emeritus, Department of Allergy, Kaiser Permanente Medical Center, San Francisco:

> You have my permission to state my position and quote me as against universal fluoridation of the water supply.[2]

Judge John P. Flaherty, Pennsylvania Supreme Court:

> In my view, the evidence is quite convincing that the addition of sodium fluoride to the public water supply at one part per million is extremely deleterious to the human body, and a review of the evidence will disclose that there was no convincing evidence to the contrary.[2]

Richard Foulkes, BA, MD (Physician). Former consultant to the Minister of Health, Province of British Columbia, Canada:

A review of literature and documentation suggests that concentrations of fluoride above 0.2 mg/L have lethal effects on and inhibit migration of 'endangered' salmon species whose stocks are now in serious decline in the US Northwest and British Columbia. Fluoride added to drinking water, 'to improve dental health', enters the fresh water eco-system, in various ways, at levels above 0.2 mg/L. This factor, if considered in 'critical habitat' decisions, should lead to the development of a strategy calling for a ban on fluoridation and rapid sunsetting of the practice of disposal of industrial fluoride waste into fresh water.[12]

Benedict J. Gallo, PhD (Botany). Research microbiologist, US Army Research, Development and Engineering Center, former teaching fellow and research associate, University of Michigan:

> The impact of fluoride on human reproduction at the levels received from environmental exposures is a serious concern. A recent epidemiology study shows a correlation between decreasing annual fertility rate in humans and increasing levels of fluoride in drinking water.[13]

Phillipe Grandjean. Professor of environmental medicine, Odense University, Denmark:

> Information which could cast any doubt on the advantage of fluoride supplements was left out by the Task Group. Unless I had been present myself, I would have found it hard to believe.[13]

Ludwig Gross, MD (Physician). Former chief, Veterans' Administration Cancer Research, New York:

> The plain fact that fluorine is an insidious poison, harmful, toxic and cumulative in its effects, even when

ingested in minimal amounts, will remain unchanged no matter how many times it will be repeated in print that fluoridation of the water supply is 'safe'.[2]

Charles Gordon Heyd, MD (Physician). Past president, American Medical Association:

I am appalled at the prospect of using water as a vehicle for drugs. Fluoride is a corrosive poison that will produce serious effects on a long range basis. Any attempt to use water this way is deplorable.[14]

David R. Hill, PEng. Professor emeritus, Psychology Department, University of Calgary, Canada:

Studies in mainstream peer-reviewed medical journals and government reports now document the fact that serious harms are associated with exposure to small amounts of fluoride – including hip fracture, cancer, and intellectual impairment. There is evidence that both individual and institutional fluoride promoters have stacked the deck, manipulated experimental results, suppressed evidence that spoke against their view, and victimised or smeared those who spoke out against them.[15]

J. William Hirzy, PhD (Chemistry and Risk Assessment). EPA scientist and senior vice-president, National Federation of Federal Employees:

Historically, fluoridation is mandated by government and rejected by citizens. Communities all over the US are currently fighting for their right to choose. Japan and nearly all of Europe have rejected fluoridation.[16]

Robert L. Isaacson, PhD (Neurobehavioural Science). Distinguished professor, Department of Psychology, Binghamton University, Binghamton, NY:

The formation of sound, decay-resistant and caries-free teeth as well as strong, sturdy bones, whether in animal or human populations, does not require fluoride, or at least not in more than minuscule, trace amounts. As acknowledged by sources cited in the report, even when a mother's fluoride intake is elevated, her milk is extremely low in fluoride, but owing to prenatal accumulation, her baby excretes more fluoride than it ingests from her milk. This fact clearly indicates that any natural physiological need for fluoride, if indeed any exists, must be exceedingly small and certainly far below that being recommended.[17]

Donald Kennedy. Scientist, Stanford University. Former commissioner, Food and Drug Administration:

> Many of the statements in the CR report on fluoridation are directly contradicted by readily available scientific research. Rather than weigh all new evidence as it appears, in a constant and critical reevaluation of the advisability of fluoridation, the promoting agencies – most notably the US public health service and the American Dental Association – have chosen to ignore any research that does not support their claims.[18]

Harold D. Kletschka, MD, FACS (Cardiovascular surgeon). Past military consultant in thoracic and cardiovascular surgery to the US Air Force surgeon-general and the surgeon of Headquarters Command, Washington, DC; Founder and first chief, USAF Cardiovascular Research Center:

> The fact that fluoride is incorporated into the mineral matrix of bones and teeth does not make it an essential nutrient. Other elements hardly considered essential, such as lead and cadmium, also accumulate in bones and teeth, and they are not regarded as beneficial. Obviously, if fluoride is *not* essential in human

nutrition, any consideration of it in terms of an 'adequate intake' is clearly not appropriate and should not be part of a 'dietary reference intakes' report.[17]

Lennart Krook, DVM, PhD (Pathology). Emeritus professor of pathology, Cornell University and New York State College of Veterinary Medicine:

> The economically most important effect of [fluoride] ingestion is decreased milk production. Milk calcium (Ca) is derived in equal parts from food and bone tissue. Fluoride is toxic to bone resorbing cells and with decreased resorption the cow does not produce Ca deficient milk but less milk in proportion to the F burden. The ideal [fluoride] ingestion is zero. Tolerance levels should be reduced to levels that protect cattle and farmers.[19]

Richard A. Kunin, MD. President, Society for Orthomolecular Health Medicine, San Francisco, California:

> Today, with so many additional sources of fluoride present in processed foods, commercial beverages, and dental care products that were not there when water fluoridation began, the total intake of fluoride, even among children has increased to as much as 2–5 milligrams or more per day, well above the initially proposed optimum of 1 mg/day (from one liter of 1-ppm fluoridated water). With these higher levels of fluoride intake, dental fluorosis and other toxic effects noted above have also increased.[17]

John R. Lee, MD (Physician), Sebastopol, California:

> No study in the past three decades has demonstrated any significant dental benefit from fluoridation. The older historical studies, on which claims of dental benefit are based, are so seriously flawed that most

independent researchers conclude they should be ignored. In fact, several recent studies, here and abroad, show that fluoridation is correlated with higher caries rates, rather than lower ones.[17]

Peter Mansfield, MA, MB, BChir (Physician). Director, Templegarth Trust, England:

> No physician in his right senses would prescribe for a person he has never met, whose medical history he does not know, a substance which is intended to create bodily change, with the advice: 'Take as much as you like, but you will take it for the rest of your life because some children suffer from tooth decay.' It is a preposterous notion.[20]

Gene W. Miller, PhD (Biochemistry and Toxicology). Former head of biology, associate dean of science and dean of environmental science, Utah State University:

> It was found that among the environmental pollutants, fluoride was most damaging.[21]

Paul H. Phillips, Department of Biochemistry, University of Wisconsin:

> Fluorine is known to be an enzymatic inhibitor which interferes with metabolism of breakdown of glucose, between the 6-carbon and 3-carbon compounds. The metabolism of glucose or its breakdown is our primary source of energy for maintaining life and doing useful work.[2]

J.J. Rae, PhD (Biochemist). Associate professor of chemistry, University of Toronto:

> It is known as a scientific fact that fluoride is a deadly poison to enzymes, upon which all life depends.[2]

Albert Schatz, PhD (Microbiology). Former professor of science education, Temple University, Philadelphia. Nobel Prize winner for his discovery of streptomycin:

> Contrary to what is widely assumed, the toxicity of fluoride is not always related to concentration. Under certain conditions fluoride toxicity actually increases as the concentration decreases. This is what is known as a paradoxical effect.[2]

Bruce Spittle, MB, ChB, DPM, FRANZCP. Senior lecturer, Department of Psychological Medicine, University of Otago Medical School, Dunedin, New Zealand:

> There would appear to be some evidence that chronic exposure to fluoride may be associated with cerebral impairment affecting particularly the concentration and memory of some individuals. These symptoms are reminiscent of those seen in the chronic fatigue syndrome.[22]

Doug D. Styne, MD (Physician). Department of Pharmacology, University of Praetoria, South Africa:

> Long-continued ingestion of minute quantities of fluorine causes disease of the thyroid gland.[2]

James B. Sumner. Director of enzyme chemistry, Department of Biochemistry and Nutrition, Cornell University. Nobel Prize winner for his work in the field of enzyme chemistry:

> We ought to go slowly. Everybody knows that fluorine and fluorides are very poisonous substances and we use them in enzyme chemistry to poison enzymes, those vital agents in the body. That is the reason things are poisoned; because enzymes are poisoned, and that is why animals and plants die.[2]

A.K. Susheela, PhD. Professor of histocytochemistry, All India Institute of Medical Sciences, New Delhi. Director, Fluorosis Research and Rural Development Foundation:

> What is the matter with your scientists that they allow your government to be so stupid? (4 October 1998, commenting on the UK government's support for fluoridation)[23]

Alfred Taylor, PhD. Biochemical Institute, University of Texas:

> The terrifying conclusion of the studies was that fluorine greatly induced a cancer tumor growth. If doctors and the public can be made aware of this catastrophe, fluoridation shall end quickly. It will someday be recognized as the most lethal and stupid 'Health Program' ever conceived by the mind of man, witch doctors and blood-letters not excepted . . . the growing weight of scientific evidence that water-borne fluorides, even at 1 ppm, have toxic possibilities must finally be recognized.[2]

Hugo Theorell, MD (Physician). Nobel Prize winner for his research in the field of enzyme chemistry:

> The fluoride ion exerts its toxic effect by inhibiting the action of many enzyme systems.[2]

Harold Warner. Professor emeritus of research, chief of Biomedical Engineering Division, Emory University Medical School.[14]

John Yiamouyiannis, PhD (Biochemistry). Recognised as the world's leading authority on the biological effects of fluoride:

> In the United States fluoridation accounts for more than 30,000 deaths a year, of which 10,000 are due to cancer, and it accounts for chronic effects in the majority of the Unites States population.[7]

Rudolph Ziegelbecker, PhD (Physician). Institute of Environmental Health, Graz, Austria:

> European scientists, in evaluating USPHS claims of fluoride dental benefits, find these supposed benefits are random, i.e. not dose-related, and are unconvincing whereas the toxicity (dental fluorosis) is dose-related.[24]

Nobel Prize winners opposed to fluoridation

Apart from three Nobel Prize winners among the names above, another thirteen Nobel Prize winners in chemistry and medicine have either opposed fluoridation or expressed reservations about it:[25]

Adolf Butenandt (Chemistry, 1939)
Arvid Carlsson (Chemistry, 2000)
Hans von Euler-Chelpin (Chemistry, 1929)
Walter Rudolf Hess (Medicine, 1949)
Corneille Jean-François Heymans (Medicine, 1938)
Sir Cyril Norman Hinshelwood (Chemistry, 1956)
Joshua Lederberg (Medicine, 1958)
William P. Murphy (Medicine, 1934)
Giulio Natta (Chemistry, 1963)
Sir Robert Robinson (Chemistry, 1947)
Nikolai Semenov (Chemistry, 1956)
James B. Sumner (Chemistry, 1946)
Artturi Virtanen (Chemistry, 1945)

Reference

1. Colquhoun J. Influence of social class and fluoridation on child dental health. *Community Dent Oral Epidemiol* 1985; 13(1): 37–41.
2. Famous quotes on fluoride and fluoridation. Leading Edge Research Group. http://www.trufax.org/fluoride/quotes.html.

3. A crack appears in the fluoride front: After surveying the growing evidence, a high-profile advocate has second thoughts about the safety of fluoride. Report by Michael Downey, *Toronto Star*, 25 April 1999.

4. Meinig GE. Fluorine could be trouble. *Ojai Valley News*, 5 January 1986.

5. Murakami T. Dose for incipient acute fluoride intoxication: True science and false science. *Fluoride* 1998; 31: 55–6.

6. Sutton PRN. Fluoridation: a fifty-year-old accepted but unconfirmed hypothesis. *Med Hypotheses* 1988; 2: 153–6.

7. Yiamouyiannis J. *Fluoride: The aging factor*. Delaware, OH: Health Action Press, 1986.

8. Testimony of Robert J. Carton before the Honorable Judge Peter Grim, State of Wisconsin, Circuit Court, Fond du Lac County, Decision and Order Case No. 92-C579. June 29, 1993, *Safe Water Association, Inc.* v. *City of Fond du Lac*.

9. Connett P. The fluoridation of drinking water: a house of cards waiting to fall. Part 1: The science. *Waste Not* #373. November 1993. Canton, NY: Work on Waste USA.

10. Diesendorf M, Colquhoun J, Spittle B et al. New evidence on fluoridation. *Aust & NZ J Public Health* 1997; 21: 187–90.

11. Erickson DJ. Mortality in selected cities with fluoridated and nonfluoridated water supplies. *N Engl J Med* 1978; 298: 1112–6.

12. Foulkes RG, Anderson AC. Impact of artificial fluoridation on salmon species in the northwest USA and British Columbia, Canada. *Fluoride* 1994; 27: 220–6.

13. Should Natick fluoridate? A report to the town and the Board of Selectmen, prepared by the Natick

Fluoridation Study Committee, Natick, MA, October 23, 1997. http://www.cadvision.com/fluoride/natick.htm

14. Leading Edge Research Group. http://www.trufax.org/ fluoride/fluorides.html.

15. Hill DR. Fluoride: risks and benefits? Disinformation in the service of big industry. Paper presented at the public forum on fluoride and fluoridation, sponsored by the Chemical Institute of Canada and CADACT, Petroleum Recovery Institute, Calgary, Canada, 29 September 1992.

16. Hirzy JW. EPA scientists take stand against fluoridation. http://www.rvi.net/~fluoride/070797.htm.

17. Letter from the University of Kansas (Chemistry) to Dr Bruce Alberts, president, National Academy of Sciences, 15 October 1997. http://www.sonic.net/ ~kryptox/nutri/alberts.htm.

18. Letter from Donald Kennedy, also signed by Paul Ehrlich, to Consumers Union, 4 March 1969. http://www.rvi.net/~fluoride/book.htm.

19. Krook L. Abstracts of papers presented at the XXIInd Conference of the International Society for Fluoride Research, Bellingham, Washington, USA, 24–27 August 1998. http://www.trufax.org/fluoride/23rd. html.

20. http://www.npwa.freeserve.co.uk/index.htm.

21. Gritsan NP, Miller GW, Schumatkov GG. Correlation among heavy metals and fluoride in soil, air and plants in relation to environmental damage. *Fluoride* 1995; 28: 180–8.

22. Spittle B. Psychopharmacology of fluoride: A review. *Int Clin Psychopharmacol* 1994; 9: 79–82.

23. Fluorides are general protoplasmic poisons. http:// www.cadvision.com/fluoride/quotes.htm

24. Ziegelbecker R. Fluoridated water and teeth. *Fluoride* 1981; 14: 123–8.

25. IFIN #218: Nobel Prize winners concerned about fluoridation. Fluoride Action Network, http://www.fluoridealert.org

Index